PATRICIA REDLICH is a well-established columnist with the Sunday Independent newspaper. In addition to writing topical feature articles, she writes a health column and a problem page for adults and teenagers. She appears regularly on television and radio programmes and has been active in a wide range of social issues in both Ireland and Germany.

While living in Germany, she obtained her primary degree from the Goethe University of Frankfurt and her Masters degree in Psychology from the Ruhr University of Bochum. After working as a psychotherapist in Germany she later returned to Dublin to take up a position as Senior Clinical Psychologist with the Eastern Health Board. Her interest in journalism developed as part of her activities in social issues and communications became her full-time occupation.

The Book:

This book is written as a guide for parents but will interest all those involved with the education and emotional development of children. It deals with children and sex education from the earliest years to teens, including the whole complex area of sexual love and the difficulties which arise for both parents and teenagers. The style is informal but the issues are faced squarely. Patricia Redlich draws on a wealth of personal and professional experience to help parents talk with their children in this crucial area of personal development.

The Video:

While the book is self-contained, the associated "Sex and Love" video has been specially prepared to give parents confidence. The video compliments the book. The live discussion was recorded by Patricia Redlich with a group of parents. The topics covered will hold your interest and answer many of the questions you always wanted to ask. This is an informative programme which will enliven the whole subject and help you with sex education, particularly when talking to your teens.

For my son Alex,

with love.

And for Val,

who created the happiness

which made the writing

of this book possible.

©1995 Quest Communications Ltd.

ISBN 0 9526819 0 0

All rights reserved. No part of this publication may be reproduced, stored in retrieval system, or communicated in any form or by any means, electronic, mechanical, photocopying or otherwise without the prior written permission of the publishers.

Cover photograph of Ms Redlich by Colm Henry, reproduced courtesy of the Sunday Independent.

Cover design by Deirdre Barry.

Published and produced by:
Quest Communications Ltd.,
3 Springfield Park, Foxrock, Dublin 18, Ireland.
Tel.: +353-1-2894455. Fax: +353-1-2898045.

Typeset by Tony Moreau.

Printed and bound in Ireland by ColourBooks Ltd.
Baldoyle, Dublin 13.

Sex and Love

Talking with the Children

A Guide for Parents

by **Patricia Redlich**

CONTENTS

Preface		xi
Chapter 1	A Difficult Task	1
Chapter 2	Soft Landings	13
Chapter 3	The Language of Love	25
Chapter 4	Embarrassment	37
Chapter 5	Privacy	49
Chapter 6	Boys	57
Chapter 7	Girls	69
Chapter 8	Homosexuality	77
Chapter 9	Dire Warnings	83
Chapter 10	Pleasure and Desire	93
Chapter 11	Birds and Bees	101
Chapter 12	Physical Changes	109
Epilogue		115

PREFACE

On reading an early draft of this book, my editor, Kate Cruise O'Brien, asked me to remember, while writing, that you needed me to be your friend.

I am. But the litmus test of true friendship is the preparedness to say the hard thing. As a friend, I have to tell you what you need to hear. Not, perhaps, what you'd like to hear.

I cannot let you off the hook. How could I, believing as I do that parents are the ones who must teach their children about sex and love? Others may help, but sex education is ultimately your concern.

It was necessary to try and sweep away the cobwebs that clutter minds, the attitudes which harden hearts, to clear the intellectual and emotional stumbling blocks that make talking with our children about sex and love so difficult.

Forget the trendy concept of feedback, which pretends that there is no pain involved in learning. Gaining new insights always hurts. It's an effort to change ideas and attitudes and behaviour. It inevitably involves self-criticism, and regret about mistakes made.

It is worthwhile. Teenagers need their parents. They will love you, and be forever grateful that you made the effort.

I do hope this book will help. And that it entertains. Sex education should also be good fun.

CHAPTER 1

A DIFFICULT TASK

WHEN my brother, Paul, was about 11 years old, my mother finally persuaded my father to take him to one side and tell him the facts of life. I think she thought he needed to know, since he was the only boy among a gaggle of girls, two of whom were now heading towards womanhood. The birds and the bees were starting to stir in our household. It seemed like the right time to do it.

She also undoubtedly wanted, albeit quite unconsciously, to avoid awkward questions from him, as we, his older sisters, started diving into bathrooms with brown paper bags under our arms, or slid down the stairs, surreptitiously heading towards the bin in the back yard.

I don't believe she communicated her reasons to my father. I've asked her, but she doesn't remember. Given this was the 50s in Ireland, the probability is that there was very little said, even in our reasonably enlightened household. My mother was undoubtedly also quite unconscious about the tactics of her timing. I'm certain, however, that she didn't expect my father to talk of periods, or the precise workings of a woman's body. She just felt it was time Paul knew something, since we older girls had been initiated into the adult world.

The conscious intention was to inform, to let him in on the secret we now shared with our parents. But, however unwittingly, it was undoubtedly also presumed that, if he heard about the birds and the bees, he'd be filled with sufficient awe at the wonderous workings of nature, that he'd hold his tongue, ask no questions about the suddenly secretive behaviour of his older sisters. He was to be informed, but also silenced, told in order to prevent him from talking about matters sexual.

My father went to bed that night, happy and self-confident, assuring my mother that Paul now knew everything there was to know. His son was equipped for life.

Next morning Paul cornered my mother after breakfast, when my father had been kissed goodbye and waved off to work on his Vespa scooter. Paul asked her if she thought there was something seriously wrong with Ben - in a brave attempt at being modern, our parents had reared us to call them by their first names. According to Paul, our father had sat him down at the fire after we'd all gone to bed and talked to him intently for two hours. Paul didn't understand one single word of what was going on, but did realise that it was something profound and very important. He wondered, he told my mother anxiously, if Ben had been trying to tell him that he was suffering from some serious illness? He was worried about becoming an orphan.

Ben had undoubtedly talked of zygotes and embryos, cell division and chromosomes, genes, gender, sperm, semen, intercourse, the endometrium and amniotic fluid. He would have been hot on biology, my father, as a largely self-educated man, and intense in his lecturing mode, by definition doomed to tell Paul nothing the child could assimilate, or even begin to understand.

No, my mother didn't then go on and explain about conception, birth, love, sex and joy. Paul, like most boys, was left to learn about the facts of life from his peers, and probably later on from his wife. Or perhaps he has remained, much like the men at my dinner table recently, in relative anatomical ignorance. He's busy making his way in Australia, so I didn't ring to ask. But the taboo about talking did work. He never asked any of his four sisters any embarrassing questions. Sex education had taught him to hold his tongue.

For the record, my mother didn't talk much to the girls about love and sex either, let alone desire, temptation, or emotional needs. We simply got the conception and birth bit, along with a general explanation about periods, since they were what prompted her to begin in the first place.

Looking back, I think of my parents with affectionate indulgence. They tried to be progressive and proper, do the right thing, prepare their children for the adult world of love and sex. It would be foolish, however, to tinge the memory with any sense of superiority. When it comes to sex education, much is still the same.

Certainly the world our children live in has changed dramatically. Scantily clad female bodies now adorn every billboard, abortion is debated in their daily diet of soaps, incest, rape and paedophilia are a regular part of the media menu, and youth culture has become highly sexualized, the body beautiful draped across just about every music video in town. On the positive side, subjects relating to sex are now dealt with in the schools. Biology lessons, talks on relationships, and programmes on the dangers of sexual abuse, alcohol and drugs, are now commonplace in the classroom. There are also some good books around, which we can hand to our older children, or talk through with the younger ones, books which would have been banned when my father messed it up with Paul all those years ago. And some of the television soaps teach our children too. They are modern morality tales.

A DIFFICULT TASK

But when you look closely at what my parents attempted to do, the particular problems they faced, and where they fell down, it's clear that not much has changed, at least not dramatically.

They were trying to open some kind of communication line with their children about one of the most central issues of our lives, namely love and sex. Of course they had to try themselves, since there were no textbooks or teachers or television to do it for them. In the absence of anyone to hide behind, they were attempting to talk to us.

Like all children, we had already eavesdropped on much of the adult life around us, still peopled 40 years ago by closely knit extended families. In our case, the eavesdropping was made easier, and potentially more extensive, by the fact that my parents didn't believe in sending children to bed, or banning them from adult company. We heard much of what was going on in the turbulent emotional world of aunts and uncles, grandparents, cousins, neighbours and friends, and were fascinated, and informed.

We knew, long before we were nine, that the lady down the road had actually been deserted by her husband, that he was not, as the official neighbourhood version would have it, simply seeking work in England. We also knew she had another man who loved her. We knew too that both our grannies, strong and fiery red-headed women, who were often angry or fuelled by irritable energy, had unsatisfactory sex lives. Our grandfathers were good men who didn't quite pass muster in the bedroom stakes. We accepted there was good reason for our grandmothers' tempers, and were understanding, rather than upset, when they gave out to us unnecessarily.

We worried too, with our elders, about the uncle who married quite late in life because of a possessive mother, felt for the friend of the family who wanted no more children and slept apart from her husband, felt protective about the aunt who lost her first two pregnancies in unhappy miscarriages, and cheered on the uncle who left a loveless marriage to run off with the woman he adored. We positively reverberated with the passion and pathos of adult life. I have no memory of anything other than an unambivalent partisanship with the hero, or heroine, of any particular family drama, and always felt my parents' sympathies were on the same side.

Of course we had no notion of what sex actually involved. We just grew through childhood recognizing that it was important, both for women and for men. Our parents, and wider family environment, communicated a fundamental emotional message. Happiness hinged on physical togetherness with a sympathetic soul-mate.

The problem, when it came to talking about sex itself, was that my parents seemed to believe they were starting cold. They didn't think of beginning with the story of the runaway uncle, or link into the aunt who

A DIFFICULT TASK

was saddened by her early miscarriages, or talk about the obvious happiness of the lady down the road, now that she was loved again. They didn't think to build on the emotional knowledge we shared, or to draw on our common history of sympathetic involvement in the lives of those around us.

Like the society they lived in, my parents saw sex as something separate, quite different from the drama of daily living, a subject quite apart from the normal chatter that endlessly went on between us. Although they had read Freud, and were committed to a more enlightened kind of child-rearing, sex itself was an isolated issue, which they could not deal with, in the context of daily domesticity.

They also made the mistake of believing that sex education, proper, was solely about anatomy and biology. Instead of delving into those feelings we already knew so much about, they isolated sex education from emotions, and talked of facts.

They took us aside, and talked to us, very seriously, about a subject-matter called the facts of life. And then there was silence.

My parents had failed to communicate. Even worse, despite their best efforts, they closed the communication channel between us on that all-important issue - sexual love. We were estranged and embarrassed by their approach, shocked by the suddenness of it all. We absorbed the unspoken message that sex was somehow different and separate, not allowed in normal social intercourse. We were left with the lonely task of trying to integrate this factual knowledge into our emotional worlds, without any help from them. Poor Paul, of course, had to try to find out what it was all about in the first place.

Surveys, statistics and what parents and teenagers say, all tell us that little has changed.

Boys are seldom talked to, and usually learn from their peers. Certainly fathers say nothing to their sons. Daughters do somewhat better. Mothers have to prepare them for their periods, so they are obliged to say something to them about sex. Fathers say nothing to their daughters either. And they are largely shut out from the world of budding womanhood, which at best is related back to them through their wives, as they chat together in bed at night.

We're not doing much better than our parents did. That shouldn't surprise us, or make us feel guilty, but merely make us determined to try and get it right. There is good reason why we're still floundering.

There was a perception abroad that our parents' generation had problems with sex, and, by extention, with sex education, because of the stranglehold an authoritarian Catholic Church held on Irish society. The basic assumption was that, once the grip of the church was loosened, sex would come into its own, all questions relating to sex solved by the mere loosening of the religious noose.

A DIFFICULT TASK

By some absurd leap of logic, it was also presumed that the sexually permissive society would effortlessly herald in a new, and uncomplicated, line of communication between parents and their children, making sex education a mere doddle.

That is patently not so, and it was mere foolishness, or helpless hoping, on our part to think it might be thus. Attitudes to sex run deeper and wider than the influence of any particular church.

The idea my generation grew up with of woman as either whore or madonna was not new. Nor was there anything unusual about the belief that sex was something which needed to be tamed, a dark force which lead to damnation, rather than the springboard for great joy and happiness. Such ideas went back to biblical times, and far beyond. The idea that women needed to be cleansed after childbirth, and hence the process of 'churching', still prevalent in my childhood, was not invented by the Catholic Church. Sex as the enemy, rather than a friend, is a theme of all ages. How could we have expected to overthrow such ideas overnight?

Younger parents today, who happily missed the repressive 50s, are still moulded by such attitudes. The shackles of sexual repression are not easily shaken off.

Sex is not simply a question of morals in a religious sense. Our attitudes to sex are not merely a question of sin, or serious transgressions. Sex is not the sole concern of religion. Sex education involves clearing our heads on many issues which are of social as well as religious concern. There is a secular morality too, and we've to make our minds up before we can be confident in talking to our teens.

How do we view births outside wedlock? Do we think they are a good idea? How do we define sexual propriety? What are our ideas about the age of consent? Should a man be allowed to have sex with a 15-year-old girl? Is marriage still sacred? Do we believe in romantic love? Do we see men as predatory sexual prowlers, or is there something in the idea of woman as temptress. If so, what do we say to our boys, and our girls, in order to protect them?

These are issues which have been debated down the centuries. They have been the subject of concern, not just for church fathers, but for governments and heads of state. Such subjects involve the social order as well as morality, are of secular, as well as religious, concern. Societies have struggled with, but never entirely resolved, the various dilemmas these questions pose.

It was naïve of us to think that once sexuality was no longer so repressed - because people had eased themselves away from the authoritarian structure of the church - all questions relating to sex would suddenly be solved.

We still have to decide what is good and bad, permissable and not permissable. If anything, our difficulties are now greater. We've done away with dogma, and now have to make decisions about everything ourselves. Our children ask us why, and we have to have a personal answer. 'Because the church says so' is no longer enough, either for us, or for them. There is an increasing emphasis on personal conscience. Nobody can tell parents what to do with any real authority or power to convince. When you think about it, we are undoubtedly more unsure than our parents were, about what exactly we wish to tell the children. We are facing the painful and difficult task of being authoritative ourselves, rather than relying solely on some higher power.

It was also naïve to think that, once we shrugged off the shackles of sexual repression, we would rise like some sensuous Phoenix from the ashes, with no scars, hang-ups, doubts or dilemmas about sexual love. Even those born much later than the harsh 50s, still carry the legacy of those unenlightened times. Attitudes run deep, and don't go away within one generation. Parents are still struggling, and quite rightly so.

It was even more naïve to think that a sexually permissive society would encourage better communication among consenting adults, and hence make talking with the children easier. Anyone who has even dipped their toe into the world of casual sex knows that the price generally paid is even poorer communication.

More, rather than less, uncertainty has resulted in

greater anxiety about saying what you really feel, or of even finding out what you really feel.

How, then, did we really expect communication with our children would be easier?

A happy sex life doesn't necessarily solve the problem. It doesn't automatically equip you with the skills to communicate about sexual love - to anyone - let alone to your children. Or more particularly to your budding teens. Even if we ironed out all our hang-ups, resolved all the emotional, moral and social questions about our own sexual behaviour, that wouldn't guarantee that we could talk to our children. Certainly, being at ease with your own sexuality and happy with someone you love, helps. But it doesn't necessarily mean that sex education comes easily.

We have got better at the early birds and bees. We talk about anatomy and biology. Or point out certain dangers. But we still find it difficult to accompany our children through their sexual development. We don't speak to them about love, desire, need, anguish, joy, responsibility and how to make difficult decisions. We don't talk to them about love and sex.

Like my parents, we leave our children alone. They still negotiate the mine-field of sexual love without the wisdom of their parents. Boys, in particular, are still singularly solitary. Fathers are still absent.

They need us on that journey into adulthood. We want to walk with them.

CHAPTER
2

SOFT LANDINGS

THE 'Safe Sex' message is simple. Sex can kill, is what it tells us. The answer is less simple. Wear a condom, is the solution offered, probabaly the best advice a general public sex education programme can muster.

Indiscriminate sex may not be good for the soul. Even Hollywood acknowledges that. Rehabilitation programmes are now run there for men and women who see their promiscuity not as pleasure, but as addictive behaviour, a problem they have to deal with. A public health education programme, however, has a difficult task. It's into damage limitation, rather than salvaging people's psyches. It just aims to keep you healthy, and alive, while you're doing whatever you choose to do.

The 'Safe Sex' message doesn't preach anything other than how to avoid sexually transmitted diseases. The only thing you have to worry about, it seems to say, when it comes to having sex, is that you avoid disease. Sex is considered solely as a question of health. Wear a condom, and the world is your oyster. Without ever formally alluding to it, the 'safe sex' message carries a moral code. It's fine to have sex, quite thoughtlessly and randomly, provided you avoid catching a sexually transmitted disease. Concern is limited to health, makes no mention of minding the heart, emotions, soul or mind.

Medicine has to be pragmatic. Think of the public uproar when doctors try to decide to do something as simple as refusing to treat smoking-related diseases until the patient kicks the habit. Or when they consider not doing liver transplants on chronic drinkers. Public medicine is not allowed to moralize. So it simply says, wear a condom, because sex can kill. That's understandable. But it's not enough for our teens. They need to hear more.

They need to hear that sex is about feelings. That sex is not just a physical act, but an emotional interaction. They need to hear that when they make love it is not just a body they have in the bed, or on the sofa, or down the lane, but a whole personality. Despite what the permissive society may say, we don't just put our pants back on and walk away, untouched by a sexual encounter. All sexual experiences shape our personalities, affect our perception of ourselves, make us feel better, or somehow diminished, depending. Our teens need to hear that.

Parents have to face the fact that sex education comes packaged in a moral code, whether it is formally expressed or not. When we talk to children about sex, we tell them what we really believe about sexual love, whether we mean to or not. We impart to them a set of values, give them a series of do's and don'ts, let them know how we believe people should behave, how the sexual relationship between two human beings should be conducted.

When parents hand over the role of sex education to others, or simply settle for putting a book on his bedside table, rather than talking to him about love, lust and how to look after the girl he likes, we are passing up a very valuable opportunity to pass on our views about sexual morality to our young ones. We are leaving it to others - the school, the media, or mere book-writers - to form our children's morals.

It seems such a strange decision to make. Sexual love is so central to our lives that it shapes our whole existence. Broken marriages, broken hearts, lost dreams of love, wreak far more havoc in peoples' lives than lost job opportunities, or exams indifferently passed, or shortfalls in the educational process. Yet we make all of those things our business, expend endless and loving concern on what happens to our children on the schooling front. And then we turn our backs on them when it comes to sexual love.

We don't default entirely, of course. Our behaviour towards each other, the views we express when something arises like a heroine in a soap getting pregnant, or the way we react to things our children do, like having the boyfriend in when they are babysitting for friends, all that allows our children to know how we feel. Our reactions to those situations are an important part of sex education. But we are letting slip a huge sphere of influence, if we fail to talk to our teens about sexual love, and settle instead for merely reacting, when they do something we don't approve of.

Parents argue that they feel left out. They'd like to be more involved with their teens, to talk to them, but feel they are not wanted. And people talk endlessly today about peer pressure, about the fact that a youth culture, rather than adults, largely dictates what our teens think, and feel, and do.

Perhaps we should wonder how that youth culture came about, and in the wondering, see how we might change things.

Isn't it possible that we *laissez-faire* parents, terrified of being authoritarian, and with no guidance about how to do it better, have left our children largely to their own devices?

Having ditched the total package of a dogmatic church teaching, perhaps we found it just too hard to work out a moral and intellectual position. It was a tall order, anyway, for just one generation. So we left it to the children to find out for themselves. More precisely, society at large started talking directly to our children, rather than through the filter of family. A separate youth culture was born. Teenagers now had a world of their own. The peer group became a point of reference, a strong influence to be reckoned with. Parents now had serious opposition in terms of telling their teens how to live.

We shouldn't feel guilty. That was what was needed. The tight structures of the family did have to loosen, in order to allow enlightenment in.

Nor is anything necessarily lost. The purpose of these reflections is not to castigate, or make people feel even more anxious. We can claw back our influence. Parents have already taken the first step. They want to. They see it as an important part of their role to help their teens by talking to them about sex and love. Our children want it too. Yes, I know teens run away when we try to corner them, but that's just embarrassment. Our job is to override that embarrassment, to take whatever opportunity we can find to open a discussion, to tell them how we feel and think. All we need to do is rein in that *laissez-faire* attitude a little. We've to start paying attention to our teens in particular. We need to muscle in, make ourselves heard, flex our authoritative muscles, gently, but firmly.

When we were both struggling to bring up sons who were bright, independent, and looked old beyond their years, a friend of mine finally threw reasonableness to the winds on the subject of her son's drinking. He was only 16, and didn't drink much. But he did manage to make the occasional visit to one or two pubs. So did mine. Having exhausted all her powers of persuasion on an unheeding head, my friend had a photograph of her son blown up to poster size, his age stamped across it like a police photo-fit, and threatened to post it up outside every pub in town, accompanied by the caption, 'This boy is underage'. She was in grave danger of going seriously over the top.

Nowadays parents feel powerless, part of the price we've had to pay for shaking off the shackles of an authoritarian society. That society underpinned the power and privilege of fathers as the head of household, and mothers as women with a will of iron, who definitely knew best. We said we didn't want that, which was fine. Now we've written ourselves out of history to the point where teenagers think they know best. Three-year-olds think they know best.

Parents feel that society is no longer on their side. We don't want our teens having sex too early. We look at the sexualized society they live in, and feel helpless to stop them. We know we can't lock them up, change the circumstances of their lives and the nature of modern society overnight. We are in grave danger of believing that we have no influence at all.

Not so. The surveys all show that teenagers not only love their parents dearly, but look up to them. They are among the people teens admire most. Teenagers also believe that parents should set the agenda for sex education. They believe we should have a real say. They want to hear from us. They say, too, that they feel comfortable talking about things that matter with their mothers, including sex. Fathers still lag sadly behind in the talk stakes, don't seem to talk to their teens about anything.

Times are changing. That's not just because of AIDS. We're all beginning to wake up to the fact that simply doing what you want, sexually or otherwise, is not good enough. We're looking again at marriage, love, and the meaning of life, taking stock of what has happened over the past 40 years. We're rediscovering words that almost went out of fashion, like personal responsibility, choice, wisdom, and the ability to wait. Teenagers themselves don't think early sex is necessarily a good idea. And they certainly still believe in old-fashioned ideas like fidelity and commitment. Parents are not as helpless as they think. The times are on our side.

My son, Alex, seldom told me anything about school until he entered second level education. I was a working mother, and didn't get home until shortly after five. By that time, anything Alex had wanted to communicate had already been discussed with his granny, whom he rang, or who rang him, most afternoons. Or had already been told to the childminder, who picked him up from school and brought him home to our house. By the time I arrived in his homework was finished. So were any questions he might have had, or things he needed to talk through about the day's happenings in school. Anything I heard was secondhand, any attempts I made to talk to him were shrugged off. He was no longer interested, for that day at least.

Small children need to communicate instantly. When there is something in their head, they want to talk. If they have a question, they want it answered, now. Sex education, like breast-feeding, should be given on demand. Older children are not much different. They can wait until tea-time, but they do need us to be accessible then, emotionally as well as practically. Adults do too.

A woman patient of mine was married to a good man. He was also a news addict, kissing her absent-mindedly on the cheek when he came home from work before before heading for the evening television news. He then tuned in the radio. And then it was another television channel. It was eight o'clock each evening before he really looked at his wife. By then, the woes of the day had hardened in her heart. She was no longer interested in letting him know what was going on in her life. The solace of his attention came too late.

My father was fond of lecturing. He simply didn't know how to give a short answer. Whenever we asked a question he felt a huge responsibility to tell us everything he knew. I liked that. I enjoyed being his intellectual partner. My next sister down was the pretty one, while I was the bluestocking. So I suppose listening to my father talk of maths, music and English prose, or expound at length on anything I raised with him, was my way of cornering a share of his attention.

The others could learn little from him. Or so they said. He pinned them down with a combination of bewilderment and mind-boggling boredom every time they approached him with even the simplest question.

Children need answers about sex which are short and to the point, sufficient to inform, and to answer the question asked, without burdening them with detail they do not want, need to know, or cannot properly comprehend.

A friend's grandson ran in to his mother recently and told her he'd just heard from the boy next door, that babies came out of a mother's bottom. Disgust written all over his face, he asked if this were true. No, his mother told him, it's not true, mothers have a separate and special passage which the baby travels through on its route from her tummy to the world outside and it's called a vagina. She left it at that, and her four-year-old went happily out to play again, perhaps even to correct his playmate. He didn't yet need to hear of semen, or intercourse, or how the baby got into his mother's tummy.

Sex education should be a conversation you and your children dip in and out of over the years. You have all the time in the world. The art of conversing includes listening, as well as telling, discourse rather than lecturing. It should be an easy and familiar interaction between individuals who like each other, a communication between equals, in the sense that what the child says shapes your answer. You hear his mind working, and tell it in the way he needs it to be said, in order to be accepted, and understood. Remember, the messenger is the message, how you say it is just as important as what you say.

Sexual love is central to our lives and something quite private. It is about feelings, rather than mechanics, about passion, loss, happiness and desire, rather than anatomy or biology. It requires intimacy. Talking about sex can only really be effective when such discussions take place in an intimate setting. Confronted with troublesome teens, it's probably difficult to appreciate how intimate our relationship with them really is. They seem like strangers. They are not, of course. We share daily domesticity, use the same bathroom, catch at least some of our meals together, and are all automatically affected when someone in the family gets ill or dies. There are a million strands which weave the web of family. This is an intimacy which runs so deep that any current crisis is merely a ripple on the surface, soon swept away. We shouldn't be afraid to approach our children. Nor should we accept it when they attempt to turn us aside. And we should definitely feel confident about putting our foot down.

SOFT LANDINGS

Sexual love is about difficult decisions. The themes are general ones, and every teenager could write the list. So could every parent. Should I approach the girl I like? Can I really believe him when he says he loves me? Does my girlfriend really mean it when she says she's sorry? How do I handle the fact that she flirts? Do I really want sexual intimacy, or what parents used to call heavy petting? What do I do about jealousy? What am I really saying if I decide to go along with a grope on the dance-floor? Is it time for sex?

The solutions, however, have to be found by individuals, our sons and daughters. And individual circumstances are always different. It's not enough to teach them general principles, like the need for proper self-respect. They need help and guidance on an ongoing basis. They also need limits, and specific instructions.

In an ideal world, that 16-year-old daughter, off next Saturday on a date with the boy she fancies, would know your feelings about proper sexual behaviour. She would be self-confident, have sufficient self-esteem to allow her to say no, if it needed saying, because she knew you cherished her. She would have some insight into how boys feel and think. She would understand, too, the kind of signals she herself sends out. And she'd be aware of her own needs. She'd be wise about how other people handle such situations. Through years of talking to you, she'd have her own sense of personal morality. She'd know how to take care of herself emotionally. She'd also be with a boy you knew, because you'd insisted on meeting him. You would know where she was going. And she'd have a deadline for getting home.

Certainly it would not be proper for teenagers to discuss all the details of their sexual behaviour with their parents. Privacy has to be respected here as elsewhere. But they do need to be able to avail of their parents' wisdom. They need a personal ear, someone who is, first and foremost, on their side, someone wise who knows them, and is available more or less on demand.

Parents are poised on the brink. They know they are needed. Their teenagers know it too. All parents have to do is gather the mantle of their courage around them and begin.

The psychotherapist Carl Gustav Jung, whose professional business was the problems of the mind, revealed in a biography that he had spent most of his life trying to dodge depression. Finally, he told his biographer, he gave in, stopped fighting, dropped into depression, and found it a surprisingly soft landing.

Parents will be surprised, and hugely gratified, once they take the plunge and start talking to their children. No, start talking with their children, about life, love, sex, and the pursuit of personal happiness.

CHAPTER
3

THE LANGUAGE OF LOVE

Teenagers titter during biology lessons. That's not because they are silly, but because they are sane. They know, without necessarily being able to formulate their thoughts in coherent language, that sex is all about feelings. Every day they deal with lust, desire, jealousy, attraction, shyness, shame, anxiety, anguish, discomfort, bewilderment, and love.

Human biology may be the physical basis of it all. But it is irrelevant in terms of daily experience. How you feel is what counts. The fact that hormones play a part is merely academic to teenagers. Obviously it's necessary to know these things, but the biological 'facts' are far removed from what they actually feel as they grapple with their sexual development. Sex as a biology lesson is somehow absurd, and decidedly beside the point.

If the lesson strays beyond reproduction, leaves zygotes and embryos, chromosomes and genetic inheritance, to talk of the penis, vagina and penetration, teenagers titter even more. Many adults do too. Sex is then being talked of as something mechanical, an erection being explained as the process of blood flowing to the penis, rather than the result of desire. But there's nothing mechanical about our attitude to sex. We don't experience it in terms of mechanics. We experience sexual love as a series of feelings, ranging from desire to sexual satisfaction, lust to loving tenderness, or sometimes - unhappily - anxiety, loneliness, disgust or regret.

A few years ago I reviewed a video called 'The Art of Loving'. It was teaching people about sex, and sexual pleasure, and it portrayed couples in various stages of sexual activity. These images were accompanied by a quiet measured commentary from two experts, who spoke in academic tones, teaching and telling while the couples cavorted. It felt ridiculous, and I, only half-jokingly, suggested that the video should be viewed with the volume turned down.

The video was fine. It just suffered from the inherent absurdity of trying to deal with sex as an academic exercise. Sensual images fed your eyes, while your ears were assaulted by technical facts. The discrepancy was disconcerting. It left me grinning.

Drawings on a blackboard are certainly not sensual. But it would be foolish if we pretended that they don't evoke erotic images, remind us of erotic feelings, require us to deal with our sexual excitement. They do. Handling this is a task which requires sophistication. So teenagers titter. Mature adults don't. If we are honest, however, all that maturity brings is the ability to talk objectively about matters which are still full of feeling. All we learn is the ability to step outside our excitement for a while, to master it while we talk, or listen. Talking academically about something as turbulent and full of feelings as sex is, is, by definition, a distortion of reality.

Sex education is not about teaching children the mechanics of sex, or the science of biology. Parents have to talk to their children, and particularly their teens, about feelings. It's a daunting task.

Parents are not entirely spared the trap of the biology lesson when they try to talk to their teens about sexual love. They, too, face the difficulty of talking about sex in the dry tones of serious discussion. But it is possible for parents to create a greater intimacy, to come somewhat closer to the world of emotions. They already have an intimate relationship with their children. The setting of the family home is less clinical than the classroom. The inherent problem of talking about sex, of setting sexual excitement aside, and talking in a formal tone is still there, however. The result is embarrassment.

The discussion about sex between parent and child is beset with its own peculiar, or rather unique, problems. Teenagers are trying to pull away from us, to establish their independence, and sex is one area where that independence is essential. Talking about it with their parents is - even in an ideal scenario - somewhat uncomfortable. The feeling of independence is threatened, the intimacy too great, the desire to get away sometimes quite desperate.

Teenagers wriggle uneasily because they are forced to acknowledge that their parents are sexual beings. Talking about sex makes that a fact they cannot avoid. Parents and children are a bit paranoid about privacy, once talk turns to matter sexual. Both are fearful that their lives will be intruded upon to an unacceptable extent. Both are busy erecting emotional and behavioural barriers, even as they speak. All of that is normal, and necessary. But it makes talking about sexual feelings a difficult task.

Even a very happy sexual relationship leaves us ill-equipped to talk to our children about sexual love. Sex is a silent endeavour. We don't have a lot a practice in talking about sexual love, not even to each other. Unless, of course, something is wrong. Then we have to learn to talk, put words on what we want and feel, discuss difficulties.

On an everyday basis, we don't usually discuss sex, in the sense of discourse or debate. Endearments are uttered when we're making love, sounds and sighs escape, the odd joking comment is made when something comes undone, there's an unexpected interruption, or you get a sudden cramp in your thigh. We may engage in pillow talk, ask our partners what pleases them most, and recall happy memories shared. Discussions, however, don't take place, not in the sense of anything that could enter the public arena. The language and the content of what we share is strictly private. It offers no basis for sex education by parents, doesn't really contain any words we could use to our children.

One of the earliest lessons I learned as a therapist was that people don't just have difficulty talking about their feelings. They believe it to be positively dangerous. It's not simply that our culture is low-key, or that we see the understatement as the highest form of civility. We have so little practice at expressing our feelings that we're frightened of them. Feelings are strangers. We have no language for them, no words.

Nor do we know how to listen when other people try to express themselves. We back off. Certainly things have improved. But it's still difficult. Ask anyone who has lost someone they love about the reception they receive, if they try to express their grief, even as little as one month later. And it's not just men who have such difficulties, although they are notorious when it comes to dodging emotion.

We are able to express anger. Unlike many of my manic depressive patients, who were only angry when mania took away any worry about what other people thought, who could only express how they felt when cloaked in the mantle of 'madness', most people are able to let rip. People say what they really feel when anger is ignited.

We learn anger at our mother's knee, hear it in our father's voice, experience it everywhere we turn. We are taught to be angry. It is socially acceptable. Rage also overrides our concern about being loved, our anxiety about rejection, our worries about offending others, and our real fear about possible dangers. Anger makes you strong - at least for a while.

In the absence of rage, it's hard to overcome our inhibitions about expressing strong feelings - except perhaps when we're drunk. Drunkenness - like mania - is another kind of 'permission'. You can subsequently distance yourself from whatever you said.

Saying soft things shows our vulnerability. To talk of love, or dependence, or sorrow, makes us feel somehow powerless, not quite in control. In our competitive world, it makes us seem less of a winner. Talking about feelings takes courage. You have to be prepared to admit you're not entirely on top of things. You have to have self-confidence in order to show vulnerability. It takes true humility. That's something we can only manage if we have true self-esteem, believe we're good, lovable, deserving of respect and proper treatment. Not many adults have got that far. Most of us have difficulty showing our soft underbellies. We are terrified that if the world sees our weakness, it will move in for the kill.

Parents have to face their own personal demons, when they talk to their children about feelings. They have to rise above them. Hopefully your journey through life has helped. Perhaps knowing that your children need to hear from you will help, give you the courage to jump, however awkwardly, into that complicated but very rewarding world of feelings. Your children do need to hear from you. They need your help in order to be happy and adjusted, not just in their sexual lives, but in every aspect of their existence.

Shortly before I left home in 1965 to get married in Germany, my father took the opportunity one evening to tell me I'd been a good daughter, and that he realized, now that I was leaving, that I'd taken a bit of a back seat in the family. I was the eldest, so I was expected to be onside, almost part of the parenting, so much always seemed to be happening to the younger ones. That's not, of course, necessarily the whole truth, and it's certainly not the way my sisters and brother see it. I had also been sick several times, and got a lot of parental attention for that. But I had always tried to keep a tight lid on my emotions. I tried hard not to be any trouble, like many eldest children. I thought my parents had enough hassle in their lives without me adding to it. I wasn't very good at saying how I felt. In the process I became emotionally invisible. That's what my father was trying to touch on before I left. His attempt left me enraged, angry at his apparent belief that one sentence would undo a lifetime of lack of acknowledgement. It took me many years to become emotionally visible again. I had to learn how to show hurt and disappointment, rather than hiding it entirely, or occasionally expressing it in a quite distorted fashion - by getting angry.

The truth is, that if you are not able to express your feelings, if you can't say what you feel, and ask that your feelings be respected, then you are truly powerless. On two counts.

If you cannot make your emotional voice heard, other people cannot really see you. If you don't clearly register your emotions, you do become invisible. That's what men, suddenly catapulted into a mid-life crisis, go through. They suddenly realize that the world around them doesn't know how they feel, doesn't see their neediness, is dismissive of their despair, worse, doesn't even hear it. It's what women feel too, when they disappear into the role of being merely mother. It's what they mean when they say that they are taken for granted.

If we cannot put words on our feelings, we cannot make them our own. If we can't express our feelings, they run amock. That can be as simple as a sudden display of terrible temper about something seemingly innocuous, when you shout and roar because a husband is half an hour late for dinner, or scream at children who spill crumbs on the floor. All the pent-up hurt about a thousand injustices which were never challenged at the time, suddenly erupts. And then you're in the wrong, yet again. You got angry 'over nothing'. It can be as serious as attempted suicide, or threats of physical violence, when someone we desire or love doesn't return our feelings.

We are not in control of ourselves if we can't reach our feelings. They master us, rather than us mastering them. That means we can neither aspire to happiness, nor properly handle distress.

Teenagers have to be able to talk and think about their feelings. Those are mighty feelings - lust, desire, jealousy, love, fierce protectiveness, deep attachment, and our teens need a lot of help. They need someone who is sympathetic, on their side, who really has their best interests at heart.

Our teenagers get into trouble about sex because of the feelings involved. That trouble can be personal unhappiness, or the lifetime commitment of having a baby, or a thousand traumas in between. That's where they really need our help, however bumbling and incompetent we may feel.

They need help even more than we did. When I was growing up, strict social taboos helped keep our feelings in check. Certainly it was brutalizing. Instead of discovering our emotions and learning to keep them under control, those sexual feelings were simply denied, dismissed, and the subject of dire threats about damnation. It wasn't totally effective either. Some girls did get into trouble, which was a fate worse than death. But the social taboos in my day, backed up by church teaching about morals, did keep behaviour in check. It did put an external control, a limit, on where our feelings might lead us. The many people of my generation who were virgins when they got married were not men and women who had no sensuality. They were afraid. Or they shared the ideals of their church. And we were not constantly reminded about sex by girlie magazines, posters, movies, or the media at large. There was no sexiness around.

Teenagers today have to deal with their sexual feelings themselves. Society no longer exerts the same degree of emotional control and suppression. That's good. But it's also very difficult. Sex education is the art of helping them. It's a big step for parents. Many don't feel that well equipped. Children are, however, far more forgiving than we realize, far more rewarding to help than we can imagine. However fumbling and awkward our attempts, provided they are done with love, our children will benefit, and be grateful. And like everything else, it gets easier with practice.

Sex education is not the unknown territory we fear. Life has given us insight. We are experienced, have wisdom. We know the feelings our teens are struggling with. We still feel them, though not as painfully, as rawly, as in our youth. Take a walk down memory lane and remember - sexual love when it's all so new and bewildering, exciting, wonderful, and full of terror. Our teens are simply repeating our experiences.

Talking is the art of listening. Create the conditions, and they'll tell you. As much as is proper for you to hear anyway.

CHAPTER 4

EMBARRASSMENT

Throughout my teens, I trudged up the long icy road to our local church each day during Lent. Seven o'clock Mass in an equally icy corrugated iron structure, stomach still empty because I was receiving the sacraments, liturgy in Latin, my missal guiding my responses, the whole process low-key, quiet, and contemplative - and physically punitive. I was skinny, somewhat anaemic, suffering terribly from the cold and tired out, trying hard, with long hours of study, to escape the poverty of a northside Dublin working-class estate in the late 50s.

I thought I was pleasing God, while my sister still believes I was into self-flagellation. Whichever, I was certainly no oddity, but very much part of a culture which thought discomfort was positive. It was seen as a rite of passage into self-discipline. Without it, there was no maturity, only people who dodged responsibility.

SEX AND LOVE

Discomfort went out of fashion sometime in the 60s. It became a dirty word. Pleading that you felt uncomfortable became accepted as good reason for not doing something you disliked. Discomfort became a legitimate excuse. It's not.

Parents see the sex education of their children as part of their proper role. When they don't do it - or fall at the first hurdle, talking only of the birds and the bees to the little ones and then staying silent - they say it's because they haven't got sufficient information. All the surveys show that parents feel they need far more knowledge - sexually transmitted diseases generally, AIDS in particular, physical development of boys, and sexual pleasure being the subjects most often mentioned. Parents are not telling lies to the pollsters, and this book, in other chapters, gives you all you need to know.

When you ask parents personally, however, they tell another tale. They don't talk to their children about sex, they admit, because they feel embarrassed. Their discomfort about the subject matter shuts them up.

Discomfort, of itself, of course, shouldn't stop us doing anything. Who actually likes changing dirty nappies? Who wants to change a wheel on the side of a wet and windy road? Embarrassment is no excuse for dodging sex education.

On the contrary, embarrassment is part and parcel of sex education. It's proper, good, the correct feeling to have.

EMBARRASSMENT

But the issue of embarrassment when it comes to sex education is far more important than that. Embarrassment is part and parcel of sex education. It's inevitable. Quite properly so.

Sex is private. Parents, quite rightly, like it that way. The horror of the noisy bedsprings, when staying over Christmas back in the family home, with Mammy and Daddy sleeping next door, still sits in our neck. That does not improve anybody's love life.

When we tell our children the facts of life, we've outed ourselves as sexual human beings. We declare ourselves lovers rather than garden gnomes, put meaning on the cries and whispers coming from our bedroom. When we talk about sex to our children, we create witnesses to our own private lives. That's disconcerting. Parents talk about embarrassment, but it's actually social discomfort. Not nice, but inevitable.

It's less trouble with the little ones. Sex for them is still, more or less, of academic interest only, a subject of curiosity rather than self-discovery. They don't understand desire, so they can leave sex aside more easily, once their curiosity has been satisfied. They may ask, just for clarification, if you do it too, but then forget all about you once they've understood the message.

Teens are different. Sexual love is beginning to loom large on their emotional agenda. They really are witnesses, sleeping next door. At the end of the day, parents must handle this as they think best. Certainly you have a right to your own love life and you would be very foolish indeed if you started to put it on a back burner, just because informed teenagers now inhabit the house. Both for your own sakes, and for theirs. We tell them most by what we do, rather than what we say. Happy, loving and sexual parents give children a model of how marriage should be, help them create the same happiness for themselves, later on in life.

That said, the discomfort is very real. Perhaps for a while you may decide to temper the level of bedroom turbulence, ditch the idea of night-time love-making only, and take advantage of the times when the teenagers are out, or use the newly enlightened household as a reason for occasionally getting away alone together. Whatever strategy you adopt, you must insist that your bedroom is a definite no-go area, even to the younger ones, unless they are in serious distress. Parents need a private world too.

None of that alters the fact that it is embarrassing, a new situation which takes time to get used to. It's uncomfortable, for both sides. There's no way of easing that discomfort, however. Avoiding talking to the children in the first place merely means sticking your head in the sand. They hear about sex anyway, in the crude and ignorant banter of the school-yard, neighbourhood road, or sports club. Far better to tell them yourselves. Their speculation about how you behave in the privacy of your bedroom will then, at

EMBARRASSMENT

least, be in the context of warmth, intimacy and love. It will be gentler, because the knowledge came from you.

A friend of mine, a doctor working night shifts, was falling into bed recently as her husband got dressed around 7 o'clock in the morning. Their six-year-old burst into the bedroom, took one look at his father's boxer shorts, and declared he knew exactly what they had been doing. 'You've been sexing', he said. His tired mother asked him what he meant, explaining that she had never heard the word 'sexing' before, which was true, but not the whole truth. She was anxious to take this opportunity to talk about sex, since she had not yet told him anything at all about the birds and the bees. Her son gave her an exasperated look, told her she knew perfectly well what he meant - which was of course the whole truth - and went down to breakfast. That evening, while she made dinner and supervised his homework, she broached the subject again. After much muttering he finally said to her, 'All right, but we'll have to leave it till later. If I told you now it would only put you off your dinner'.

Talking to our children about sexual love is also embarrassing because of the reception we get. We're telling them about something we feel is important, sensitive, and very central to our lives. They very often react with disgust, dismissiveness, and, particularly if they're older, with the deep and obvious desire to get away from us as quickly as possible. That's not just discomforting or embarrassing. It hurts.

It helps to see the children as hapless, rather than actually passing judgement. The young ones don't understand desire. They are not yet clued into adult sexual pleasure. They haven't got the emotional and intellectual capacity to completely understand. Outside the framework of desire, sex must seem rather ridiculous. If you don't understand sexual need, and no small child does, imagining intercourse could put you off your dinner. Or at least make you despair of the sanity of adults. That's not a judgement. We've no need to feel defensive. He cannot understand because he's too young.

Teenagers do understand, however imperfectly. An important part of adolescence is learning to handle rapidly developing sexual desire. Their disgust, the way they strain at the leash when we try to hold on to them long enough to talk, is an attempt at self-defence. They use disgust as a barrier. That barrier is not just between them and us, but between them and their own emotional turmoil.

Teenagers are beginning to feel adult sexual excitement. That's hard to handle, changes everything utterly. Boys are now the opposite sex. Girls are objects of sexual desire. Bodies are something to catch a glimpse of, arousing emotions which are difficult to contain, which makes it hard to stay cool, or appear sophisticated and sure. Curiosity is intensified by sexual interest. Bodies no longer behave themselves. Uncontrollable erections happen at embarrassing moments. Talking in class to the boy who, only recently, was merely a mate can lead to arousal so fierce that it's positively uncomfortable. Expressing disgust is a way of keeping a lid on such sexual excitement.

Young teenagers still haven't completely cut the emotional umbilical cord either. They are still going through the emotional process of transferring affection from their parents onto members of the opposite sex. Once children have reached the age that affection becomes sexualized, they are reaching towards adulthood. Their relationship with their parents must change. They have to put some distance between themselves and the adults they love most. They are striving, instinctively and quite unconsciously, to avoid any emotional incestuousness.

It's not forever. Just until they get their new emotions under control, and make the necessary emotional transition from the family into the outside world.

Embarrassment is not just a discomfort which we have to take in our stride because we're adults. It is not a sign of weakness, incompetence, or failure on our part - or on the part of our children either.

Embarrassment is quite proper, normal and appropriate in the context of sex education. Certainly it shouldn't last forever. And it definitely shouldn't stop us talking about sexual love. It simply signals important truths which we need to recognize if we want to give our children the correct message about sex.

Embarrassment, in this context, is actually propriety. It's the guardian angel sitting on our shoulders as we try to find the right way to talk to our children - and teens in particular - about sexual love. Sex is essentially private, part and parcel of a deeply intimate interaction. It happens behind closed doors. It's a delicate and sensitive task to talk about it.

We are also easing our children into emotional independence, when we talk to them about sex. We are telling them about something we can never share. Our relationship is changing, becoming more formal, even as we speak. We too are quite instinctively avoiding any emotional incestuousness. The very intimacy of the parent-child relationship, which helps us give the right message about love and sexual desire, is being dissolved while we talk. It takes sensitive handling. Not much different, really, from the gentle way in which a father hugs his daughter, while firmly - although non-verbally - making it clear that she's now too old to sit on his lap.

Embarrassment is the word we use. What we mean is that we tread carefully, somewhat fearfully. That's not wrong. It's right.

EMBARRASSMENT

Embarrassment is also the word we use for our hesitation in telling children about sexual love at all. Our life experience tells us that sexual attraction is a mine-field, means broken hearts, lost lives, great heartache, as well as great happiness.

We think of the telephone calls that never come, the cutting words that mean the end of a relationship, dates where no one shows up, girls who dance with other boys and leave a son standing helplessly on the sidelines, boys who promise love and take virginity, before heading out into the hills.

We think of the anguish of loving and losing at 16. We remember the viciously competitive girls who take pleasure in a hapless 15-year-old's unhappiness because her bosom is too small. We think of the difficulty of saying no, the perils of saying yes.

Then there are the husbands who don't come home, wives who are cold. Loneliness for men and women when love doesn't work out. We don't want this for our children. Looking at them, we wonder about telling them at all. Of course there are joys. But it is an unheeding hand which doesn't stay, just for a second, before it initiates children into the world of sexual love.

The reason we should go on is because we want them to be equipped for life. They need us to tell them facts, and, more importantly, to talk to them of feelings. All parents want to smooth their children's path, help them from hitting serious rock bottom, even though we know we can't shield them from all hurt. We also hope to create individuals who are capable of happiness, take life in their stride. That's why we want to tell them.

Embarrassment shouldn't stop us. It's only discomfort, nothing serious, certainly no satisfactory excuse for dodging. And no, you don't have to walk icy roads on endless Lenten mornings to equip yourself with the emotional stamina. Just accept that your feelings are quite understandable, and plough on.

There is much which will help lessen the distress. And in this book I'll tell you about language and timing, give you information about homosexuality and about how to help girls to say no. I will discuss privacy, which comes next.

For now, however, just one handy hint to ease the embarrassment.

Talking to our children about sex means we 'come out' as sexual human beings. They now know we have a sex life. That's inevitable. But it does not follow that our sex life is the proper subject of debate, discussion, or any kind of explanation. It is not.

Your love life is private. Your children don't need to know anything about it at all. There's no need for you to feel that, once you tell them the facts of life, they'll have the right to start confronting you with questions which you won't be able to dodge. Certainly they might be bold enough to make the odd comment. But you can stop them dead in their tracks, provided you feel confident about your right to privacy. You can be funny or stern, as circumstances dictate.

You deal with the problem best by being discreet in the first place. When you talk about sex, you simply leave out any reference to yourself. Mothers and fathers should not be used as personal examples. The most important example you give them is non-verbal. It's about the way you treat each other. That teaches them much that they need to know about how people who love each other behave. Grown-ups who disport themselves with civility, politeness, sensitivity and affection towards each other, teach their children without trying.

Remaining silent about our own sex lives limits embarrassment. It also teaches children an important lesson about intimacy, and proper behavioural boundaries. Children belong inside the circle of loving family, but very definitely outside the closeness of parental sexual love. That's something they need to know.

CHAPTER 5

PRIVACY

My son Alex was three years old when we adopted him. He had a lot of catching up to do. A kindly and loving, but very strict and rather regimented, orphanage meant he had never seen anyone cooking, or any girl, or woman, going to the bathroom. The female anatomy and nature of hen's eggs were of equal fascination to a bright mind struggling to comprehend the world around him.

I can still see his blond head bent over the cooker as he stood on a stool beside me in the kitchen, his big brown eyes nearly falling out of his head as he realized that scrambled, boiled and fried were all variations of one particular food-stuff, which started off in a shell. I remember, too, his father's well-articulated unease, as I allowed Alex into the bathroom with me, to discover how women really went to the loo.

It was, of course, all very sudden. His history and circumstances made him hungry for experience, needy for knowledge. He wanted to know. And I wanted him to know, since he was shortly entering kindergarten, that although he was born elsewhere, we were, very definitely, his parents.

Having a baby from the beginning is, of course, much easier, in terms of teaching children the facts of life.

Sex education ideally is a conversation you and your child dip in and out of, over a long number of years. It is also a relationship which moves slowly, almost imperceptibly, from uncomplicated and total togetherness, towards respectful, although very loving, physical, emotional and intellectual distance.

At every stage of that relationship, privacy plays a pivotal role. Not just in the context of sex. The journey towards healthy adult independence is a series of steps, where parents and child move away from each other. We leave and come closer, leave and come close again. We always remain their parents. With a bit of luck, we become friends too.

By the age of nine or ten or eleven, Alex was effectively shut out of the bathroom again. Not because of any pre-laid plan. I simply realized one day that a budding young man, rather than a child, was cleaning his teeth at the wash hand basin beside me, while I was under the shower. From then on, the bathroom door was always firmly closed. Nothing was said. That period of our lives, where we could occasionally chat together while we washed, was over.

PRIVACY

There wasn't a total ban on all forms of nakedness, just an acknowledgment that he had moved on.

I can't tell you when such decisions should be made. I don't even remember what age Alex was. It doesn't really matter. Children develop at different speeds anyway. Parents just need to be tuned in. All I can tell you - as a general rule of thumb - is that by puberty, such propriety should be in place. Physical privacy should be respected.

I was a psychologist, supposed to be some kind of expert. Yet all I could do was trust my own feelings about Alex. There is no formula, not even in the textbooks. At the same time we have to be careful. Instincts can be trusted, but only up to a point. We have to think too. I had three sisters and a brother, and my parents were together. But Alex was an only child. And I was divorced. That had to make a difference. I couldn't just assume that the relatively uncomplicated intimacy involved in the rough and tumble of a larger family, which was my experience as a child, was automatically appropriate for a mother and son, living alone. A very loving, but absent father was not necessarily enough to redress the balance. I had to be thoughtful, and careful, for the sake of my much-loved son.

Some parents have had it tough as children. Their parents may have been too strict. Or they may have been careless. Drink can result in serious impropriety. Our instincts, shaped when we were young, have to be tempered with reflection.

SEX AND LOVE

Think about physical violence. Some of us were physically beaten, by parents or educators, when we were small. Although we reject any idea of following in such footsteps, we sometimes still have to consciously stay our hand, deliberately walk a distance away, resist the temptation to lash out. There is no need for this to frighten us. In that split second between instinct and action, as a psychoanalyst friend of mine put it, civilization is born.

It's no different when it comes to recognizing a child's right, and need, to increasing levels of privacy as he gets older. All we have to do is stay sensitively tuned in.

There's no need to be afraid. We don't just get one shot at it. We have a million opportunities to learn the art of balancing nurturing with recognition of a child's need to independence. Privacy isn't just about matters sexual.

At some point quite early on, I gave up rummaging in Alex's schoolbag. For a while I believed that a dutiful mother should remove the rotting apple from among his books, take away the mouldy breadcrusts, empty out the collection of stones, chestnuts, pencil ends and endless scraps of paper. Then I began to realize that I was rummaging in his private life. There were notes from his teacher he didn't want me to see. Sometimes he succeeded, because teachers, too, forget. There was also - occasionally - other children's property, a problem they largely sorted out among themselves. And the odd stolen penny, as he struggled to learn about private property. I had no right to know the contents of his schoolbag. I was also relieved to relinquish the disgusting task.

As children get older, we respect the privacy of an odd dirty underpants, the accident that happened because they waited too long to come in from play. They take their own clothes to the clothes basket. As boys enter teens, we really don't want to know about their bedsheets. Their bedroom becomes their responsibility. Letters and telephone calls are private, as are the stories they tell their grannies, or the secrets they tell each other. Girls gossip, and shut their mothers out.

Privacy, in other words, is not just physical but also emotional and intellectual. Our children have to be allowed feel and think differently. Parents sometimes have difficulty with that idea. Some mothers want their daughters to always be on their side, to feel as they do. Some fathers get annoyed and angry if their sons think sport is rubbish, when they are fanatical football fans. They are suspicious if their sons like reading, while they themselves are rugger-buggers. He hates it, when he votes Tory, and his son sympathises with Greenpeace.

An older and very dear friend of mine tells the story of how he and his wife used to line up their six children to be washed every Saturday. This was shortly after the war, baths had no running water, and the scene was something akin to a busy production line. He washed the children down, while his wife dried them, and helped them into their pyjamas. One evening, my friend suddenly realized that his eight-year-old eldest daughter was not comfortable taking her place at the head of the queue. He never washed her again.

Nearly 50 years later, his voice is still full of regret that he didn't anticipate his daughter's need for privacy, didn't spare her that moment of embarrassment. Self-castigation is, of course, quite unnecessary. It was enough that he recognized her wishes so quickly, and responded so swiftly. She's lucky to have such a good father. We can't always anticipate our children's need for privacy.

Privacy allows decorum, and proper separateness, between parents and their children. It should match our children's increased awareness, march apace, as sexual knowledge deepens. If we get it right, our children will be resolutely heading towards relative independence in their thinking, feelings, and personal behaviour by the time they reach their teens. They will still need guidance, firm discipline, authority and rules. But that measure of independence will enable them to deal with their emerging sexual excitement, without either withdrawing too violently from us, or nestling too close.

PRIVACY

Privacy is a prerequisite for proper independence. It's an essential building block in the process of reaching real adulthood. The right to their own thoughts, feelings, and sphere of activity, is slowly granted to our children by an increasing awareness of their need for a private world, which parents have the courage, and self-discipline, not to enter. Emotional, intellectual and physical boundaries between parents and their children are essential. Parents and children have to be able to declare no-go areas and keep each other out.

That respect for our children suits parents too. It's easier to talk to independent minds. If they've managed to become strangers in a proper sense, while still being our much-loved children, then talk of sexual love comes easier.

Desire, lust, love, passion, and the power of sexual attraction are what our teens need to hear about. The birds and the bees are merely the beginning, facts and the mechanics of sex no more than a foundation for the knowledge and insights they really need to acquire. It is the emotions involved in sexual love which create real havoc and happiness. Talking about those adequately, and successfully, requires a certain formality in the relationship between parent and teen. Proper recognition of privacy makes that formality possible.

It is never too late. You can begin at any time. Are you still making his bed? Or dictating precisely what she should wear? Or allowing your bedroom to be randomly invaded in search of hair-dryers, soothing cream for pimples, or bedside alarm clock? Stop it, step back, and create conditions for real discussion. Then start talking. Our teens need, and want, to hear from us.

CHAPTER 6

BOYS

I went to secondary school in the centre of Dublin city, a long bus ride and even longer walk away from home. My granny, however, lived on a different bus route, not far from the school and cooked me dinner every day. She loved to have her studious granddaughter come in to eat. I loved the peace and quiet and individual attention of a meal laid out just for me. I also loved the boy I met on the No. 24 bus.

He lived around the corner from my grandmother. And, after lunch, I used to walk up the road and stand leaning against a high garden wall, waiting for the bus. I stood there, even when it poured rain, ridiculously early, pretending I didn't know what time the bus would be there. These were the days before traffic and the buses were always on time.

He was sometimes there ahead of me, which was wonderful, sometimes a little late, which was terrible because I had to wait. We stood several yards apart, leaning against that same wall every day, and didn't speak for weeks. Then we started to talk tentatively about school. But that was all. Once we boarded the bus, he invariably sat several seats in front of me on the top deck. At each bus-stop both his school-friends and mine joined us, slowly merging into one big noisy group.

He was beautiful, darkhaired, oliveskinned and blueeyed, slim, and with fine sensitive hands. I was far too lacking in self-confidence then to dare believe he might like me. Yet looking back, he must have. The fact that he stood in so many showers of rain should have told me something. The fact that I stood in so many downpours should have made him more daring. It didn't. Later on a girlfriend of mine, one of that noisy bunch on the bus, wooed and won him, and broke my heart.

Boys are in a very hard place. Perceived as teeming testosterone, threatening the possibility of pregnancy, or at least of sex too early and, with it spoiled youth, they spell trouble for parents. Yet they are largely ignored when it comes to sex education. Nobody talks to them. At best, people seem to think that age will modify their moody lust, the passing of time cover their savage breasts with some kind of civilization, or the influence of a virtuous girlfriend make them good. Their vulnerability goes unnoticed.

They face this hostile press largely alone. Certainly nobody's arms are around them. Whatever physical affection they may have got in earlier years has long since dried up. Boys hew out their manhood on very rocky ground.

Manhood itself is very hard to achieve. Our society demands a lot from men. They are still expected to be tough, to fight our wars on the battlefield or in the market-place. That's difficult enough. But we want warriors who also have soft hearts and gentle hands. Men who can care for the baby and fight off the enemy. Men who are bold enough to initiate all sexual encounters, yet subtle enough to read the signs when we wish them to desist. A tall order for young boys, struggling to become competent adults.

Our sons are needy human beings, who desire and deserve information, affection, guidance and support just as our daughters do. How could we think otherwise? How can we even begin to think of sensible sex education if we ignore boys? They are, after all, the other half of most sexual relationships.

Mothers don't make that hard place any easier. The hand that rocks the cradle still treats boys very differently to girls, and from quite an early age. We may say we hanker after "new age" man, but we still support the social dictum, that boys should be tough, or at least tougher than girls.

Boys are not comforted. Girls are. When boys come crying because they have fallen, been bullied by a playmate, or been scared by some experience, we don't hold them close as we would their sisters.

Instead we tell them not to be so silly. And we do that from the age of about three, when that babyish round softness starts to leave their lovely bodies. We insist they toughen up when they are mere toddlers. And then we stop hugging them. By the time they enter their teens, they are on their own.

When my son Alex first came to live with us, he was fascinated with my hair clips and insisted on wearing them, sometimes two on either side of his head, sort of propping each other up, because his hair was very fine and they fell out easily. He was proud of how he looked. He was so new to all things domestic that I didn't have the heart to tell him that a three-year-old boy shouldn't really wear women's hairclips. In the orphanage there were no girlie type things hanging around the boys' bathroom. He was just experimenting.

I couldn't tell Alex the hairclips were wrong. He would have thought I didn't approve of him. The relationship still felt too vulnerable to withstand that. I stayed silent. So did his dad. A few days later he started kindergarten, complete with hairclips. That evening they were replaced tidily on the bathroom shelf, without comment.

Parents cannot run totally counter to prevailing social norms, even when they want to. Schools, kindergartens, and the street, still wield great influence. Society gets its message across. That said, we do have a certain leeway in our treatment of our sons. We can still comfort them, while teaching them strategies for solving their own problems, be affectionate and warm, while easing them into independence, be gentle in our judgement, when they simply cannot cope, happily allow them to lean close to us when they really need the comfort. There is still a world of difference between macho and real male. Parents can help their sons explore that difference. All they need to do is see their sons' vulnerability, even when it's buried beneath the boorishness of emerging manhood.

Oedipus is not just a figure of Greek mythology, or the figment of a Freudian mind. Boys do have to leave the comfort of their mothers' arms. They have to take a long, lonely walk across the sexual divide, move away from the world of women and into the world of men, take on the male identity.

Any mother lovingly tuned into her son knows that at some point she has to push him gently away. She senses how he yearns to be a caring male towards her, the love and tenderness of the boy merging with budding manhood into a powerful and, for the mother, very rewarding - if not, indeed, rather tempting - combination of gentleness, deference, dependence, love, and fierce protectiveness .

Wise mothers respond when their sons start to distance themselves. Quite small boys refuse to be kissed at the school gates. Even young ones can go stiff with embarrassment at something as simple as a goodnight hug, once friends are around. Mothers quite rightly acquiesce, even though they know that what motivates their sons is society's demand for the strong silent man, which their sons are picking up, however subtly expressed, from the greater world around them.

Sex stereotyping serves an important emotional function, helping sons to wean themselves, metaphorically speaking, from their mothers' breasts. So we have to stay silent sometimes, even when we're not particularly impressed by what's happening to our sons, the attitudes they adopt, the things they think and say, the exaggeratedly male way they sometimes behave. Good mothering takes great tact. And all of us have learned that we can't use our children as weapons to change society overnight. Girls still get pretty dresses, and boys their action games and guns.

My nephew, at 11, still walks unconcernedly down the street, his small hand held happily in mine as he talks about the world, school, science, and religion. His brother, only two years older, cringes uncomfortably at even the most fleeting attempt at a hug, palpably still needing the affection, but awkwardly shaking it off.

Boys start distancing themselves even faster, and more radically, as adolescence ushers in adult sexual excitement, lust, and sexual love. They have now turned their attention towards girls, walked away from their mothers, discovered the opposite sex. Quite rightly so. But the price they pay is physical - and emotional - and intellectual - deprivation, as mothers and sons inevitably part company.

Fathers have already disappeared. The taboo about physical affection in our society hits fathers hardest, particularly when it comes to showing affection to their sons. Men are not encouraged to be affectionate among themselves. And while they may be wonderful with the babies and young toddlers, they seem to back off systematically as the children get older and reach the age of reason. Then fathers, at best, become their intellectual guides, an emotional bulwark, and of course source of funds, but they are not physically affectionate or close to their children. This is particularly the case with their boys.

This happens to a lesser extent with girls, part of it quite properly so. Oedipus plays a role here too. Fathers need to be watchful and wean their daughters gently away. But with boys there is the added dimension that affection between males is not encouraged in our society. Some would say that this is part of a collective angst about homosexuality. Others argue that it's social convention. Or part of the process of forming our boys into tough men. Whichever, the taboo exists. And boys suffer. They leave their mother, the warmth and affection of her encircling arms, and join the men, where there are no loving arms at all.

SEX AND LOVE

From the time they pull their hands away from ours as we walk down the street, to the time when they find the happiness of being held by their first girlfriend, our sons are without comfort, affection, or physical closeness.

We don't talk to them either, about the massive changes going on in their bodies, minds and hearts. Instead, we view them with a degree of hostility, or, at the very least, with incomprehension. Our sons spend the five most formidable years of their lives, largely on their own.

Boys are in a hard place.

Teenage boys can be difficult. They are suddenly big, hugely clumsy, awkward, self-centred, moody, full of rage and silly helplessness. They have gigantic feet and smelly armpits, pimples and few social graces. They don't all fit that description. But everybody knows someone who *has* a son like that.

In an attempt to be sympathetic, parents try to see them as walking hormones, physical development gone out of control, anatomical time-bombs waiting to go off.

Certainly the onset of puberty is triggered by the brain which sends messages to the testes to begin producing the male hormone, testosterone. As you can read in the chapter on the 'Birds and Bees', that male hormone is also responsible for the physical changes taking place in the boy's body, including increases in growth and body weight.

BOYS

It would be very wrong, however, to see unrequited lust as the sole reason for his moods, or hormones as the explanation of all annoying social behaviour in teenage boys.

At 11 or 12 they can still run for help, at least to an older brother. By 15 or 16 they are expected to handle all street situations on their own, square up to danger, and come home bloodied, but unbowed. Certainly their parents can no longer go out to sort out their battles. They are, in large measure, out in the world alone.

In those same short few years, they begin the struggle of learning to understand long-term consequences. They start to study for examinations which are years away, begin to eat food which will keep their bodies healthy for life, slowly start coming to terms with the fact that what they do now, matters for the rest of their lives. They may not yet think of a baby nine months down the road when overcome with lust, but they are struggling with the task of seriously deferring pleasure for long-term rewards. At least that's what we expect of them, and they are trying to fulfill our expectations.

In the meantime they have to cope with their unpredictable bodies. It's not easy to suddenly have huge feet. They have to try not to feel too anxious as they sexually develop. Boys endlessly write to me about the size of their penises. Girls can admit they're worried when a bosom develops late, or too early, but boys can't talk to each other, or to their parents. They worry on their own.

Boys feel frighteningly out of control. This body of theirs now responds with involuntary erections when they see something sexy. Lustful thoughts wander at will through heads which should be more concerned with the road ahead, the teacher in the classroom, or the maths in the book propped up on the desk in front of them.

They are also busy in that sphere which it is no longer fashionable to mention. They are trying to work out their personal moral code, trying to reconcile ideals with the demands of the real world. They are trying to decide what they really believe in. Some of that is already written in stone, their conscience already well formed as they took on board their parents beliefs, or developed what Freudians would call a super-ego. Now, however, they are trying to temper that with the new information coming in to them from the world, as their intelligence becomes increasingly independent. And they are trying to integrate their rapidly developing libido into a code of conduct that they can live with. This doesn't sound like the average adolescent, seen from the bird's-eye view of a parent trying to cope. But it is going on.

Boys are busy. And very lonely. Nobody seems to love them during these years. Certainly there is no physical comfort. Both parents seem emotionally distant. Boys dimly understand that society sees them as a

BOYS

hormonal mess. They have no clue about how to become this gentle warrior that same society seems to demand. More importantly, they haven't a notion what girls really want, or how to express their own needs.

Boys are terribly needy, lost without the kind of companionship girls and women take for granted. When they try to get close to girls they are not just doing so out of uncontrolled hormonal urges. They want affection, physical closeness, alleviation of the awful loneliness of being a teenage boy.

Boys don't look for sex just because testosterone is coursing through their veins, or because of uncontrolled lust. Boys seek early sex because they are adrift, cut loose from the family, alone.

To help them wait until they are old enough to handle a proper, responsible sexual relationship, parents need to start talking to their sons. Not just about the birds and the bees, but about everything that is going on in their heads. They also need to comfort them, be as affectionate as they can. Less criticism will give our sons more self-confidence. Praise will swell them with proper pride. He'll then be less needy, won't need so desperately to prove himself, or find a girl to say he's great. Tucked more cosily into the warm and approving bosom of the family, he'll be in less of a hurry to have sex.

CHAPTER 7

GIRLS

I left the nuns after my Intermediate Certificate. I was tired of being put down. There was enough criticism going on at home from a very exacting father. Honours in all subjects and a serious placing in the top twenty in Ireland in mathematics finally stiffened my backbone sufficiently to say stop. I knew what they were trying to do. The head nun had told me often enough. She was saving my soul from the sin of intellectual pride. That same intellectual pride gave me the credentials, and courage, to walk out, two weeks into the first term in 5th year.

I went to a vocational school and was welcomed as a person worth having, which was wonderful. I was introduced to co-education which was even more wonderful, and fell promptly in love, again. I was not quite 16.

A marvellous priest, far ahead of his time, took us for civics class once a week. He was a film and music buff and had the wisdom and courtesy to treat us as serious human beings. My intellect was now encouraged. This was my first taste of real education, as opposed to schooling for exams - as I saw it anyway - and it was magic. He talked, too, about relationships and sex. In fact, looking back, that was probably the real purpose of those classes, although it didn't seem so at the time. Sex education as a subject didn't exist then.

I was flattered and enthralled by the way that priest talked to us. But I did not like his message for girls. In fact I rejected it out of hand. Basically he said that saying 'no' was our responsibility. It was our duty to mind, not only our own morals, but boys' morals too. I was disgusted. Here was a progressive priest, whom I really liked and admired, giving me the age-old Eve as temptress routine. The man who talked to us about the impact of Frank Sinatra on music and modern pop culture, who discussed Marlon Brando and method acting, asked our opinions on James Dean and perceptions of modern youth, was now peddling the double moral standard of a society we were seeking to emancipate ourselves from. Men's sexual transgressions could be forgiven, were not really their fault. Fallen women were condemned both as sinners, and occasions of sin. We were expected to resist, for the boy's sake as well as for our own. Good behaviour was up to us.

Looking back, I don't remember feeling actual sexual desire. But I do remember the terrible anger I felt at that priest's message. That wasn't just an intellectual position on my part. Undoubtedly the strength of my feelings was some part of a battle which was already going on in my unconscious. I think I was worried that I was about to find it hard enough to be good myself, without trying to make sure my boyfriend was good too. I did love him, with all the intensity and romance of a teenager fed on Hollywood.

Undoubtedly my analysis of that priest's position was true, at least up to a point. With hindsight, however, I can see that he was trying to tell the truth. Whatever way we may feel about it, or how we think things should be in an ideal world, the reality is that saying 'no' is still largely up to girls. Little has changed.

Little has changed in our hopes or aspirations either. We may be gentler, and more enlightened, when girls get into trouble, or teens experiment too early with sex, but we don't want it to happen. Parents want their daughters to wait. All that's changed, perhaps, is the reasons we give. It used to be because we saw sex outside marriage as a sin. That was enough, covered all our concerns, was a blanket, absolute position and we didn't have to think any further. We may still have our religious beliefs. But we now have other concerns. We want our girls to wait until they meet someone who is nice to them. More precisely, since most boys are very nice indeed, we want them to wait until they are old enough to handle the intimacy of sex gently, with responsibility, and due care. We want to protect our daughters, and sons, from casual, emotionally brutal, or unthinking sexual activity. We really do want them to have the white dress, kind husband, loving wife, and wedding. We want them to be loved and cherished. We also want them - boys and girls - to have a decent education, a real chance to explore life, a chance at independence. We want them to be happy. We don't want them to have sex too early.

That decision is still up to girls. That's not because boys are bad, which they are not, or because they are driven by their hormones, which they are, but only up to a point. It's because boys are emotionally needy, and try to find consolation and comfort, as well as sexual satisfaction, by pursuing girls.

Saying no is still difficult. In fact it's more difficult because there is no longer any clear social consensus that early sex is unacceptable. The idea that sex should wait until marriage has effectively disappeared. The current moral norm is serial monogomy. That said, in Ireland at least, there does seem to be a consensus that sexual intercourse should wait until teens are around 18. Teenagers share that view.

Girls are under pressure. They cannot simply say to boys, as my generation could, that having sex is against their conscience, or church teaching, and be sure the boys will understand. Boys in my day might have argued, or pleaded, but they didn't think I was old fashioned, or some kind of sexual freak. They knew, and accepted, that I was normal when I said what they expected to hear. Not so today.

Teens are surrounded by commercialized sex. It's harder these days to forget our sexual needs. How can anyone shut out all those images? Youth culture, a modern and quite recent phenomenon, sets our teens apart, outside their parents' lives and sphere of influence. It allows them to think and feel that their lives are quite different from ours, that they cannot possibly learn from us, that only their peers can tell them how to be. It's not that black and white, of course. Teens do think their parents are wonderful and love them, want to hear from them about life, love and the pursuit of happiness. Parents are not as helpless as they feel. But they do have to compete with a teenager's peers.

Girls have difficulty saying no, not just because of boys. They have to say no to themselves too. And it's hard for them to deal with their own neediness. Sexual desire is part of it. There's also the need to be loved, thought well of, and a boyfriend offers that. The anxiety of losing him can be a powerful incentive to have sex. A young girl loves her boyfriend. She sees his neediness. Very often she feels she is the only one who sees it, because his parents are blind. She wants to comfort him. And sex is very comforting. Concern and aching tenderness at a partner's vulnerability are not feelings which are exclusive to adults. Girls want to hold their boyfriends close and console them. Saying no means fighting these feelings, as much as any sexual advance from the opposite sex.

They need wisdom and far-sightedness, not qualities we associate with the young. That's why they need our guidance.

We have to accept and understand their neediness. Then help them deal with it, without letting them get themselves into difficult situations, or allowing them endanger their long-term interests. Early pregnancy is not the only hazard. Girls run the very real risk of putting their education to one side, in the pursuit of early love. They kiss goodbye to economic independence, turn their backs on personal success. They need protecting.

Girls have to fight off sexual attention. That means they must be very self-assertive. Self-assertion is not just a question of saying no. It's about self-esteem. If a girl feels good about herself, she doesn't have to barter sex for affection. How she feels about herself is our business.

I was the eldest daughter, the bluestocking, the studious one, the brains. My next sister down was the beauty. I was competent and clever. She was competent and female. That was my father's decision, the way he treated us. Or so it seemed to me. A hard taskmaster, he made me use my head. For that, I am eternally grateful. But he didn't cherish me as a daughter. I was, at best, a companion of the mind. Ann was the beautiful one.

Girls need to feel beautiful. It is central to their self-esteem and self-confidence to believe they are attractive. And *yes*, that does mean that they need to know they are attractive to the opposite sex.

Her father is the first man in a girl's life. He's the first male she flirts with. If fathers cherish their daughters, they will be self-confident as females. They will have the self-esteem of confident young women. They will believe in themselves and their own self-worth. They won't desperately need some gangly youth to tell them they are beautiful. Properly treated by their fathers, they will go on to expect good behaviour from boys, and later on from the men in their lives.

Not everyone, of course, has a father. And some fathers don't give their daughters what they need. That doesn't mean those girls can't make it. Children have a unique capacity to soak up what they need, wherever they find it. There are always uncles, grandfathers, friends of the family, school-teachers, who will do instead. For me it was my grandfather, my father's father, who thought that I was beautiful, and precious. Certainly he was proud of my academic achievements. But only up to a point. All he wanted of me was what I already was, his beloved granddaughter.

Teenagers have succeeded in chasing their parents out of their social lives. *Laissez-faire* parents colluded in that process. Fathers and mothers hesitate to intrude. If we are serious about helping our daughters say no, then we have to change that. Your daughter's world, her girlfriends and boyfriends, need to see that she is not adrift, but a cherished and integral part of a family which cares. She needs to know it too. How you do it depends on circumstances. She also needs to be able to use her parents as an excuse, to say that they won't let her do certain things, to help her avoid what we used to call occasions of sin. She won't be grateful, of course, but she needs it.

My generation of parents started off by ditching authoritarianism. That was right and proper. For a while, parents got away with dithering about what they should put in its place. Our daughters force us to face up to the answer. We have to be wise, authoritative, balanced, sane, loving and prepared to take a stand. We have to exercise good authority.

Our daughters have taught us that parents, too, must learn to say no. Tread softly, for you tread on their dreams.

CHAPTER 8

HOMOSEXUALITY

WHEN I was about 16, a friend of mine organized a night's stay-over in a convent in town, roughly once a month, where the Blessed Sacrament was exposed 24 hours a day, and a constant vigil was maintained. Patricia got together a group of us and we did the night-shift from seven in the evening until seven the next morning. Those who were involved after ten stayed the night. It was usually a Friday night, which left us free to roam the city on Saturday morning.

We were devout and happy to do something good. The real attraction, however, lay in the night's fun. Two shared each hourly vigil, one leaving the church a few moments early to call the next two, this process going on all through the night. So did the story telling, and horseplay, discussions and practical jokes. Sleep largely eluded us. One or two of us were in love, but none of us had boyfriends. It was very much love from a distance. We had no clear heterosexual credentials. We had a wonderful time.

In today's worried world we would be scrutinized carefully, both by parents and peers. We'd be worried ourselves about whether or not we were lesbians.

Same-sex friendship is becoming somewhat suspect, which is very sad. Boys in particular are suffering a crisis in their sexual identity. And parents are feeling worried and unsure about what to think or how to behave. Given today's world, that's not surprising.

It was inevitable, and right, and proper, that as our society became more enlightened, we would be gentler about the subject of homosexuality. People should certainly not be judged, or discriminated against, or cast out emotionally or socially, on the grounds of sexual orientation. In fact, in many ways, unless you're actually looking for a sexual partner, someone's sexual orientation should be of no real concern. Why would you want to know, unless you were sexually interested in him, or her? What matters is whether or not people are good friends, reliable work colleagues, honest and honourable citizens.

That's true, but only up to a point. The reality is that sexuality is not something totally separate from our personalities. It is part and parcel of who we are, intimately interwoven into the way we behave, and how we interact with others. So of course people are interested. And of course homosexuality becomes apparent as we get to know someone, unless it is painfully and damagingly repressed. That's only as it should be.

The problem is not that we have become more enlightened. The problem is that we have a very superficial understanding of homosexuality. That often makes us ignorant and crude. It also makes us frightened. We can no longer ignore the reality of homosexuality, and we're floundering.

We're not helped by the fact that some gay activists have pushed the politics of sexuality too far. What started out as an attempt to combat prejudice and inequality has become something akin to a crusade for the gay way of life, as though it were the only real way to be. Gay politics, deliberately or otherwise, defines people in terms of their sexual orientation. Gay activists understandably set out to emphasize the positive side of homosexuality. Many now try, however, to make homosexuality trendy, not just something to be taken as given, but to be aspired to. That does homosexuals no favours, leaves parents worried and young teenagers confused, and ignorant banter the norm in school-yards everywhere.

Teenagers need their friends to validate the experience of growing up. It's like swapping stories about what it's like to be a budding woman, or an almost man. They are more comfortable in their sexuality when they have same-sex friends to let them know they're fine. It doesn't all happen with words. It's like playing on the same team. Just hanging around together allows them to share experiences, to see others handling the same situation, to learn that it's alright, whatever way they feel.

Parents always wanted to make sure that boys were proper boys and girls were proper girls. Sissy was a term of derision and girls were only allowed be tomboys until they were about seven. With the advent of gay politics, and the apparent media glamorization of homosexuality, parents have become positively jittery. Some young teenage boys, in particular, are terrified. We need to steady our nerve, and help our teenagers not to be afraid.

Homosexuality is the preference for a same sex partner. It has nothing to do with the way a man or woman looks, the things they are interested in, the professions they prefer, the way they walk, or talk, or think about things in general. The vast majority of homosexuals are not camp, or butch. They are indistinguishable from their male and female colleagues. If they tend to gather in a certain profession, for example the theatre, that's only because the theatre world has traditionally been more enlightened about sexuality. It's not because some professions are automatically gay professions. A boy wanting to be an actor, or dancer, or costume maker, wants just that. It is not a statement about his sexuality.

Homosexuals don't necessarily dislike anything either. Homosexual women like nice clothes, babies, and female chat. Homosexual men like football. Girls

HOMOSEXUALITY

who don't like pretty clothes are not automatically lesbians. Boys who do not like contact sport simply don't like contact sport. It is not a statement or indicator of their sexual orientation.

Gentleness should not be suspect in our teenage boys. We said we wanted men who were more approachable emotionally, didn't we? Why should we now worry because our boys are not macho, clumsy or loud? Men have been protesting that they're fed up with the stiff upper lip, the pressure and responsibility of constantly seeming strong and capable. Why would fathers worry, then, when their teenage sons still cry? The fact that strong-minded girls can now pursue independent careers is a measure of how much we've moved on in terms of equality. Why on earth should we be concerned at that tough teenage daughter? The typical male homosexual is just as likely to be some John Wayne lookalike, a lesbian, that beautiful long-legged blond sitting at the bar, who agrees with every word you say.

The reality is that the vast majority of teenagers turn out to be heterosexual. It is very much the norm. It therefore makes sense to stop worrying about outward signs that mean absolutely nothing, and simply presume heterosexuality. In so doing, we can be reassuring to our teenage boys in particular, who are most vulnerable when it comes to questioning their own sexuality.

SEX AND LOVE

They are frightened because they are being forced to ask themselves questions about their own sexuality, questions to which they have no clear answers. They are asked to defend their heterosexuality before they have any clear notion of what that entails. They don't know whether the fact that they like home economics means that there's a question mark over their own maleness. Society can frighten them if it asks them too many such questions, challenges their motivation for too many things they do, worries them about who they are, before they have had a chance to cement their sexual identity, to feel confident and secure about it.

Parents need to support their teenagers by reinforcing their confidence. To do that, parents themselves need to feel confident about the fact that some teens are late developers. A boy of 15, who is not yet really interested in girls, is normal. A certain amount of horsing around with their own sex is normal. Having deep, abiding and quite exclusive friendships with other boys is normal. And in this day and age, even being worried about being homosexual is normal, not necessarily any indicator that a teen is actually gay.

Parent need to jettison their own prejudices, which assume that gays look, think, or act in any particular way. They have to accept their teenager's developing personality, without fear.

Certainly some of our teens will turn out to be gay. But that will only emerge in the fullness of time. If and when it does, you will support and love them. Meanwhile relax, and reassure your youngsters.

CHAPTER 9

DIRE WARNINGS

Parents are preoccupied with sexually transmitted disease, particularly since the advent of AIDS. Any time they are asked about sex education, or what they feel teenagers should hear, or what they themselves need to know about in order to talk to their children, they inevitably mention sexually transmitted disease, put it quite high on their list of topics for sex education.

Certainly parents need to be informed about the world, need to know what's happening out there. But it's hard not to suspect that this parental interest is driven by something other than a mere thirst for knowledge. Parents, I believe, secretly hope that sexually transmitted disease, particularly AIDS, will work as some kind of apocalyptic stop sign. Parents are hoping that the threat of AIDS will put a stop to their teens having sex. It won't. Dire warnings don't work.

SEX AND LOVE

Hell and damnation didn't stop us. My generation got a single, consistent message from all sides - school, church, family and society at large. We were told that sex before marriage was a sin. We may have wanted it, felt even in our hearts that it was right, but we believed it was wrong. All the forces in our world worked against early sexual experience. A girl stood to lose everything, including the chance of Heaven. Hell and damnation played a role, reinforced the message, but that's all it did. On its own, it would not have worked either.

The message that 'sex can kill' is the wrong way to learn about sex. It doesn't work as a deterrent either. Stark health warnings about dire consequences do not have the desired effect. Anyone who doubts that only has to look at the growing statistics about youthful smoking. Ignoring 'stop' signs is not, of course, a behavioural phenomenon exclusive to young people. But it is particularly true of our teens. Hearing that they may die, on its own, doesn't stop them doing anything, let alone something as pleasurable as sex.

I talked to my son Alex about this book and, in the course of the conversation, about parents and children generally. He told me I had been a paranoid parent. He said that I had always believed he did things I wasn't happy about solely to make my life difficult. The truth, he said, was he did them for no reason at all other than that he wanted to.

DIRE WARNINGS

Teenagers don't do things according to some master plan they've worked out in detail. They haven't got some grand design for any aspect of their lives. The first sexual encounter, or any particular sexual encounter, is not the result of a systematic siege. It happens because of opportunity, because of desire, out of great emotional neediness, because society has lifted the total taboo on early sex. It happens because teenagers have no absolute belief that it is wrong. Sex happens because they give no thought to the long-term consequences, don't think beyond the moment.

Picture the scenario of a 15-year-old girl, babysitting her baby brother, with parents who think it's fine for the boyfriend to keep her company for a couple of hours, munching crisps and drinking coke in front of the television. She's too fat by current fashion standards, has low self-esteem and not too many friends. He's 16 and, like many boys, is quite desperate for affection. And they are in love.

What role could the spectre of sexually transmitted disease possibly play in this scenario? How could such a dire warning possibly act as a deterrent?

It has absolutely no relevance whatsoever. How could either of these youngsters have a sexually transmitted disease? Unless of course he or she is sharing needles as part of a drug habit and she is on the game to get the money. That is of course a problem for some, and a very serious problem too. But sexually transmitted disease is simply not a reality for most of them.

Say they were older. Say she was 16 or 17, and he was a 21-year-old Lothario, with numerous notches on his belt, and the scene was his car after a disco. Does any parent really believe that she'd worry about disease? That it would stop her making love? Change the scene again, and make him 35, with perhaps some experience of ladies of the night on trips to Thailand, as well as many ex-girlfriends. Even if that daughter knew all about it, which she probably wouldn't, would she stop?

Teenagers believe danger will never happen to them. In our happier moments, we call it the optimism of youth. Which it is. Their preparedness to take chances pleases or displeases only in the context of whether or not we approve of what they are doing. Our problem is not that they dismiss danger. Our problem is that they are not selective in the dangers they choose to dice with. In other words, they take chances we wish they wouldn't. There is, however, no Solomon who can decide where optimism ends and mere foolishness begins. In other words, our teens are not always wrong, and we are not always right.

That said, parents are quite right to wish their teens would postpone serious sexual involvement until they are old enough to take on all the responsibility involved. If we want to help them do that, we should, in a sense, forget about sexually transmitted diseases, since they are simply a relatively unlikely doomsday scenario, and one which will not stop them sexually

DIRE WARNINGS

experimenting too early.

There is much that parents can do to help their teens avoid early sex.

Temptation is something we all understand. We know how difficult it is to think of anything, let alone the long-term consequences of our behaviour, when sexual desire takes over. We find it difficult. Think how much harder it is for our teens. It takes toughness, character, self-confidence, courage, and lots of practice, to say no to ourselves, let alone to someone we love.

Parents should seriously consider rehabilitating something as old fashioned as the concept of chaperone. Why leave our teens in situations which can be hard to handle? No, we can't always avoid it. We can't follow them everywhere they go. Nor should we try. But we can make more of an effort to make sure we minimize the moments of temptation. Just as we need to lock up the drinks cabinet, or monitor the contents carefully.

Perhaps there's something you can do about that daughter's fatness, help her feel good about herself so she doesn't binge. There is certainly something you can do about her low self-esteem. You can praise her a lot, criticize very little, and only about specific issues. Don't tear her whole personality to shreds. And be warm and affectionate. That way she'll be less needy for her boyfriend's approval.

You can help that 16-year-old son too. Try to

understand how isolated he feels without any physical affection. Show him and tell him how much you love him. Praise him, and criticize only when you absolutely have to, and then more by way of telling him how to, rather than giving out to him for getting it wrong, whatever the 'it' might be.

A friend of mine tells the story of her younger brother's best mate, who was going out with his girl for years. They all moved around in the same crowd. Then she became pregnant and had a baby. He was 18, had absolutely no financial prospects, panicked, and emigrated. They had been very much in love, and neither found happiness. It wasn't that the bad one got away. He married very unhappily, had no children, and divorced. She never married and died young. He later got to know his son, but only from a distance as the child was brought up by his grandparents. He never became a proper father, is still childless.

Teenagers don't need dire warnings. They don't heed them anyway. They need reality fed back to them on an ongoing basis. They need to hear about real life. You have to talk to them about what happens when people become seriously sexually involved.

All these stories are not, and should not be, negative. They need to hear the good stories too. They need to know that love can conquer adversity, given half the chance. You should tell them about how wonderful it is when sexual love comes accompanied by real respect, proper responsibility, and true love. They need something to aspire to. Ideals move teenagers, motivate them, in a way that danger never can.

I bought a christening present for a friend's grandson recently. The lovely girl in the shop told me she was shortly to be married in the church where, as a young teenager, I used to stand and watch the brides as they came out the church doors and paused at the top of the steps, surrounded by family and friends, their arms safely tucked into the bridegroom's, their white dresses long and beautiful. It was the steps that mattered most. Twenty or more deep granite steps, stretching the width of the church portal and beyond, making every wedding regal and full of magic. The bride and groom would walk down slowly, while the whole world applauded with their eyes, allowing us onlookers a glimpse of happiness, glamour, romance and love. When I was young early sexual experimentation was forbidden. But we *were* encouraged to believe in romantic love. Those church steps made any kind of waiting worthwhile.

Parents do, of course, have to be informed about sexually transmitted diseases. Here is a short summary for you, all you really need to know in terms of conversation with a teen.

• • • • •

Chlamydia is a micro-organism which causes pain on passing urine and a discharge from the penis in men. Women may have a vaginal discharge or no symptoms at all. It can lead to pelvic inflammatory disease in women, which can in turn lead to infertility. This infection is treated with antibiotics.

Gonorrhoea is one of the longest known and most common sexually transmitted disease. It causes inflammation of the mucous membrane of the urethra in men, which results in pain when passing urine and a discharge from the penis. In women the first sign is a yellow vaginal discharge, although many women with the disease have no obvious symptoms. The infection can spread to the womb, Fallopian tubes and ovaries, sometimes causing infertility if left untreated. It too is treated with antibiotics.

Genital Herpes is caused by a virus, herpes simplex II. The virus cannot be killed, the attack clears up after about two weeks, but futher attacks can happen. Tenderness and tingling and itching are the symptoms, followed by blisters, which can become painful sores. It is infectious during attacks.

Genital Warts appear on the penis, or at the entrance to the vagina and cervix, or around the anus. They are often not noticed and can disappear of their own accord. They are also removed by application of a lotion or by surgery, but tend to recur. There is a possible increased risk of cervical cancer among women with genital warts.

DIRE WARNINGS

Non-specific Urethritis is the most common sexually transmitted infection, most often affecting men who will have the pain on passing urine and discharge from the penis as in most other genital infections. Women may have a slight vaginal discharge. It too is treated with antibiotics.

Pubic Lice, which look like crabs but are tiny, live in the pubic hair and cause itching. They can also be contracted by sharing bedding and towels. A special insecticide lotion is required to remove them.

Syphilis starts with a sore which is painless. It heals after a few weeks but the infection remains in the body and develops. Antibiotics are again the treatment used.

As you can see, the symptoms of various sexually transmitted diseases are the same. And some of the symptoms, for example vaginal discharge, can be caused by other conditions, which are not sexually transmitted. It's important to have symptoms checked out early.

Finally, AIDS, the condition which really woke people up to the dangers of sexually transmitted diseases. AIDS is the abbreviation for Acquired Immune Deficiency Syndrome. Basically it means that the human being's immune system deteriorates to the point where he or she can no longer fight off infection, and people then die. It is believed that it is caused by the HIV virus, Human Immunodeficiency Virus, which enters the cells of the body and remains there, while the immune system tries to control it. If the immune system loses the battle, the individual starts getting a variety of illnesses and is said to have AIDS. HIV is found only in bodily fluids. Of these, blood, vaginal fluids and semen are the only ones which have been shown capable of transmitting the infection.

Do remember. Our teenagers don't need lectures on sexually transmitted disease. They need stories about love.

CHAPTER 10

PLEASURE AND DESIRE

I finally got kissed in the back row of the Grand Cinema in Fairview, on Dublin's Northside. I was 14. He wasn't the boy I'd loved and lost on the No.24 bus, but one of his school-friends, whom I grew to like a lot. We never really went out together. We were always in a crowd, couples pairing off only to snog, in the cinema, away from prying eyes.

I don't remember the actual kiss at all. But I do remember the way my whole body was suffused with excited pleasure at the feel of his breath on my neck. And I remember the excited happiness and contentment of having his arm around my shoulders, long before it was clear he would ever make it to the kissing stakes. Being close was enough.

Parents feel daunted by teenage sexuality partially because - in the terminology of psychoanalysis - we're phallocentric. As a society we tend to define sex solely in terms of what happens to the penis. We see sex and intercourse as interchangeable terms. We associate sexual pleasure almost exclusively with penetration.

That's not some kind of chauvinist male conspiracy. We are quite right to be concerned about what happens the penis, quite right to see penetration as important. It's plain foolish to pretend that human sexuality has no basis in biology or to deny its function as potential procreation. Intercourse leads to babies, sometimes, so of course it matters. Human sexuality is still very much propelled by instinct, and that's right and proper.

Sexual intercourse brings great pleasure, brings a wonderful closeness and great peace. So it is not accurate to define sex solely in terms of penetration. That's a narrow, unimaginative and inaccurate way of describing it. Human sexuality involves much more.

When I give talks, I often begin by asking the audience to suspend judgement. As a favour to me. I don't mean they are to abandon their critical faculties. I don't want to brainwash, or win them over with some kind of evangelical message, gaining a gateway to their emotions by getting them to ditch all conscious thought. I just ask them to suspend that inevitable 'but' which we carry around in our heads. I ask them to postpone their reservations until they hear what I have to say. Not very different from asking our teenagers, as we regularly do, to please stop seeing us as parents, just for a moment, and listen to what we're trying to tell them. It means lifting the curtain of our prejudice.

PLEASURE AND DESIRE

The psychological story is that when babies are born, they are intensely attached to their mothers. This intense attachment is instinctive, it's about survival. There is no distinction between love and need. It's called the narcissistic phase of development, and it is open to misinterpretation. Narcissism is usually seen as simply self-love, total self-absorbtion, preoccupation with one's own body. But that's not quite correct. The baby's interest does, very definitely, extend to his mother. He does love her. But he does so under the illusion that he's the centre of the universe and she's a mere appendage. Self-love sees others all right, but as flunkies and slaves.

This is acceptable, and necessary, in babies and young infants. All of us can identify with that. Think of how frightening it is, even as an adult, when we contemplate the idea that someone we love dearly is a totally independent person, who can withhold the love and attention we need if he, or she, so wishes. It is painful to realize that we have no real control, but only need, and the hope that our beloved will go on loving us. How much worse for babies who cannot even survive physically without us? They have no way of independently moving on to someone else. That's why it's so essential that small infants' needs are met, immediately.

Rearing infants up to toddler stage is very much a question of loosening that umbilical cord, to allow the dawning, and painful realization, that *they* are the dependent ones. We have to help and guide them through their own individual Copernican revolution.

As the small baby develops, zone after zone of its body is energized with sexual pleasure and delight, starting, predictably, with its mouth. This process travels right throughout the baby's body, including the sphincter muscles and urethra around the age of two, the genitals and the whole musculature of the body. Swinging on a swing is a sensual pleasure.

As the child becomes genitally sexualized, he or she goes through the Oedipus phase. The child, quite unconsciously, begins the process of coming to terms with the fact that he has to move on, away from his parents, that it is not proper or appropriate to be that close anymore. This is the time when the child realizes he is not all-powerful, not the centre of the universe, that he does not possess, or own, the nurturing adults around him. They are quite separate human beings. He's a separate human being too. He sets out in earnest to become totally independent. Temper tantrums are par for the course.

At puberty, the hormonal changes, triggered by a message from the brain, mean that children start developing adult sexual characteristics, breasts, body hair, the rapid development of sexual organs. Their sexual feelings are awakened, enter their conscious thought. Such feelings are now, at least potentially, manageable. The body is fast becoming adult. The mind is becoming independent. The emotional bond between parent and child loosens rapidly. Sexual love is now possible.

Our teens are not just desperately seeking sexual intercourse. They are seeking all the comfort that sexual love brings. In a very real emotional sense, they are attempting to recreate that wonderful closeness they had when they were infants. This is not a sign of immaturity. It's the way we adults are too. Teenagers want and need physical closeness. They need to be at one with somebody else, to have someone who understands completely, who is totally on their side. They have to learn that such symbiosis is not possible, or only possible up to a point. Once adult, we are inevitably individuals, and hence, by definition, separate.

Teenagers experience their sensuality right throughout their bodies. Touching is hugely pleasurable. Holding hands means everything. Hugs full of affection are heaven, even the gentlest kiss true paradise. Babyhood pleasure at being held and touched is rekindled, with a vengence.

Sexual excitement is also felt in the genitals. Boys have involuntary erections. Girls' vaginas become moist with dclight. Both sexes have involuntary orgasms. But our teens are not tunnel-visioned about sex. They don't see it, experience it, or even desire it, solely in terms of penetration.

They may, of course, learn to do so very fast. They will learn our tunnel vision unless we abandon it. It's time we did so anyway. We no longer accept the biological message, backed by much of traditional church teaching, that sex is exclusively about procreation. Why, then, should we see sex solely as penetration?

Teenagers may see intercourse as a necessary rite of passage into adulthood, feel they have to do it in order to be grown up. They are in danger of narrowing their own sexual experience, ignoring all the other sexual pleasures they get, seeing them as second-best, compared to this all-important act of intercourse.

We have to help them avoid that trap. We have to try and create an emotional environment which helps them wait, be content with the stage they are at, and leave sexual intercourse until later.

Sexual pleasure involves the whole mind, body and heart, has a thousand ways of expressing itself, is the joy that puts that special spring in our step. It fulfills emotional, intellectual and physical needs. It encompasses our entire being. In a very real sense, it is indistinguishable from sexual love. The happiness it brings lies not just in what we get, but what we give. We have rescued what's best from that infantile joy, and added to it the sheer bliss of sharing, of loving somebody else. Not for what they give us, but for what they allow us to give them.

We say teenagers suffer from puppy love. That's a serious, and quite inaccurate put-down. They are, indeed, like puppies, but only in the sense that they show us so unashamedly how lovely and joyous and physically pleasurable it is to love somebody else.

That's the story. Like all stories, or theories, it's just one way of trying to get at the truth. Hopefully it offers some kind of working model. You will, of course, do with it what you please, believe what you choose, or see fit. That's all anybody can do. The story has succeeded, however, if it softens your heart, and gives you the confidence to guide your teenagers with a tender, yet firm, hand.

CHAPTER 11

BIRDS AND BEES

Sitting at a dinner party several months ago, I asked where exactly, in a woman's body, did conception take place? Where was the egg when it met the sperm? I was, of course, thinking about this book.

Nobody knew. Six couples, with 15 children between us, and we had no clear idea. The men knew little about a woman's anatomy, were hazy even when ovaries were mentioned. They reverted to jokes, not exactly out of embarrassment, but more as a tried and trusted means of dealing with the subject. The women had the technical jargon, were prepared to discuss the subject seriously, but knew they were only guessing when it came to where it all began. As it turned out, we all guessed wrong.

The egg is fertilized as it makes its journey down the Fallopian tube. But I will begin at the beginning. Most particularly for men, so they can stop joking, and start talking seriously to their sons.

During intercourse, around 500 million sperm pass through the penis into the vagina. They swim into the womb, or uterus, through its neck, called the cervix. The cervix is full of mucus, with only a small hole to allow periods through, but at the time of ovulation the mucus thins to facilitate the sperm's passage through.

Having crossed the womb, the sperm then swim up the Fallopian tubes, although only a couple of thousand get this far. If this happens around the time of ovulation - an egg can be fertilized for between 12 and 24 hours after ovulation - there is a mature egg already in one of the Fallopian tubes. The sperm surround it. They release an enzyme which dissolves the covering of the egg and, all else being equal, one of the them finally penetrates the egg and fertilizes it. When this happens, no other sperm can get through.

The fertilized egg, called a zygote, then continues on a four-day journey down the Fallopian tube, enters the womb, floats for two or three days, and then attaches itself to the lining of the womb, the endometrium. It is at this site that the placenta, which transmits nutrition from the mother to foetus, begins to grow. The amniotic sac, a bag of fluid which cushions the baby also forms. The womb keeps its lining. No periods occur. The woman is pregnant.

At the point of fertilization, thousands of genes, containing information from each partner's genetic background, meet each other and create pairs of genes. These genes are contained in chromosomes, and human beings have 23 pairs of chromosomes, rod-shaped bodies found in every cell in the body. The egg contains 23 chromosomes which pass on genetic information from the mother, and the sperm contains another 23 chromosomes, containing the genetic information from the father, which then pair up in the new life being created. Genes determine, or help determine, things like hair colour and body height, as well as certain inherited illnesses such as haemophilia or health conditions such as the predisposition to asthma or allergies.

One and a half days after fertilization, while the egg, now called a zygote, is still on its journey down the Fallopian tube, the egg has split into two connected cells. This is the first of a series of divisions which create the billions of cells which make up the body, each cell containing those 23 sets of chromosomes, or full genetic information.

About seven days after fertilization, the ball of cells has a hollow space at its centre. This structure floats in the womb for several days and then embeds itself in the lining of thc womb. It is now an embryo.

Scientists say that conception is a process, beginning with the fertilization of the egg in the Fallopian tube, and completed when it finds its home in the endometrium, or lining of the womb. Theologians, however, may disagree. They say that conception happens at the moment of fertilization.

SEX AND LOVE

Once embedded, the embryo develops quickly, so that eight weeks later it has a humanly recognizable form, with face, limbs and all the major organs. From now on in it is called a foetus and will be born about 40 weeks after the woman's last period.

Labour begins when the uterus, or womb, starts to contract. The contractions then increase in intensity and frequency. As this happens, the cervix, or neck of the womb, dilates, opens wide enough to allow the baby travel through. The amniotic sac, containing the fluid which surrounds the baby during pregnancy bursts, and the fluid passes out through the vagina.

The pelvic girdle is the ring of bone involving the hip bones and lower spine, which are held together by strong ligaments. During birth, the baby has to pass through a narrow opening in that pelvic girdle. This is made possible because hormones are released during pregnancy which relax the ligaments. This, in turn, allows the pelvic girdle to become wider and more flexible, sufficient to give way as the baby makes his or her way down, usually head first and facing backwards, through the vagina, and out.

At this stage the umbilical cord, which is a feed line from the baby's belly button to the placenta, is still attached, and the placenta is still inside the womb. The cord is then cut, the placenta delivered down the same route as the baby, and the process is over - more or less. A baby is born. You can decide whether to talk to them about the pain, exhaustion, and sometimes

BIRDS AND BEES

the necessity to have the vagina cut and subsequently stitched, depending on need, and medical orthodoxy.

Pregnancy can, of course, be avoided. But don't use the following as a personal guide to perfect family planning. All I'm doing is summarizing, solely for the purpose of a non-specialist talk with your questioning child.

To begin with, if you don't have sex, sperm never enter the woman's body. It's called abstinence. The sperm never get a chance to make that long and hazardous journey in the first place. Withdrawal before ejaculation has the same effect, if it works. So does wearing a condom. They both prevent sperm entering the vagina even though you've had intercourse.

The diaphragm or cervical cap, usually used in conjunction with spermicidal jelly or cream, allows sperm into the vagina, but prevents it from getting any further. The cap covers the cervix, preventing entry into the womb. Spermicides are just that. They kill or disable sperm.

Couples can also avoid having intercourse around the time of ovulation. This is somewhat controversially called the 'natural method'. It means that sperm may make it to the Fallopian tubes, but they don't meet an egg, because the woman isn't ovulating. The contraceptive pill contains hormones which prevent ovulation in the first place, in other words attempts to ensure that there's never any egg to meet, at any time of the month.

The IUD, or intrauterine device, once called the coil, is inserted into the womb. It either stops the sperm passing properly through the womb, on their way to meet the egg in the Fallopian tube. Or it can make the womb uninhabitable, make it impossible for the fertilized egg to find a nestling place where it can grow. The 'morning after' pill contains hormones which have the same effect. They prevent implantation, to use the technical phrase.

Finally, male sterilization involves cutting the sperm duct, or vas deferens, which runs from the testes to the penis, thus preventing sperm from being released. Female sterilization involves cutting, or blocking, the Fallopian tubes, meaning the egg doesn't go anywhere either.

Sometimes pregnancy doesn't happen, despite our best endeavours. This failure to conceive can be inexplicable, since no obvious cause can be found, leaving even the scientifically orientated medical experts wondering whether emotions might not also play a part in the whole process of becoming pregnant.

Sometimes the difficulties clearly lie with the woman. Problems range from failure to ovulate to blocked Fallopian tubes or infections such as Chlamydia, a sexually transmitted disease, which can leave women infertile.

BIRDS AND BEES

Men may have very low sperm counts, or be completely sterile. The sperm themselves may be poorly formed, or have problems making that long journey from the vagina to the Fallopian tubes. They may also lack the ability to penetrate the egg when they meet it. Or both partners may also be suffering certain nutritional deficiencies. Zinc, for example, is thought by some to be very important for healthy sperm.

You now have the knowledge, and the technical terminology. I'm not suggesting that this is the way to tell it to the children. Quite the contrary. My father did, and left my brother Paul clueless. This will prevent you from being floored when the whiz-kid has his first biology lesson and tries to use science as a means of dodging discussion.

CHAPTER 12

PHYSICAL CHANGES

Parents ask for information about changes at puberty. They do so, not out of academic interest, but because they want to reassure their teens. Parents are right. Those teenagers badly need that reassurance. What follows is some detail about male and female anatomy, the menstrual cycle, male reproductive system and the changes that take place as our children become teens.

There are about 400,000 eggs present in a girl's ovaries at birth, although only around 400 will ever be used. Her reproductive organs lie protected within the bone structure of the pelvis. The womb lies in front of the rectum, above and behind the bladder. She has two ovaries, one on either side, each with a Fallopian tube running from it into the womb. The womb's neck, or cervix, leads into the vagina.

The vagina is a muscular passage leading from the cervix to an opening in the external sexual organs known as the vulva. The walls of the vagina are elastic and stretch open during intercourse. A membrane called the hymen partially blocks the vaginal opening in young girls, and this membrane can be torn, or stretched, by vigorous exercise or by the use of tampons, as well as actual sexual intercourse.

The vulva consists of two outer fleshy lips, called labia, on which the pubic hair grows. Inside these are two thinner and hairless lips also called labia. Between these you find the clitoris, then the opening of the urethra, which leads to the bladder, and then the larger vaginal opening, leading to the womb. Unlike boys, girls have a separate access to the bladder and their urethra is much shorter, part of the reason why women are more prone to bladder and kidney problems such as cystitis. Infections have only a short journey to travel.

Girls - as well as boys - also have a pituitary gland, which is central to sexual development.

The pituitary gland is an egg-shaped structure, consisting of two sections divided by a clear line of cleavage and attached by a stalk to the base of the brain. It is known as the master gland of the endocrine system, or the conductor of the endocrine orchestra, since it secretes hormones which affect the whole glandular system of the body. It also produces hormones which influence the growth of the body. And it affects the development, and ongoing functioning, of the sex glands.

PHYSICAL CHANGES

At the onset of puberty, a signal in the brain kickstarts the pituitary gland into action. In girls, the gland then releases specific hormones - follicle-stimulating hormone (FSH) and luteinizing hormone (LH), which stimulate sac-like structures called follicles in either one of the two ovaries.

The follicles in the ovaries then swell and release the hormone oestrogen, which causes the lining of the womb to thicken, ready if needed for a fertilized egg. One particular follicle contains the ripening egg, and is the only one to mature completely. About half-way through the menstrual cycle, this follicle swells to the point of bursting, and releases a mature egg. This is called ovulation.

Once empty, the follicle closes up again and starts producing the hormone progesterone, which stimulates the blood supply to the lining of the womb. In other words, it helps to prepare the womb to receive a fertilized egg.

The egg travels down one of the Fallopian tubes, which run between the ovaries and the womb, and if it doesn't meet and mate with sperm both it, and the empty follicle which once contained it, disintegrate. This results in a rapid dropping off of levels of oestrogen and progesterone, which in turn causes the lining of the womb to be shed through the vagina. The cycle is up and the girl has her period. This happens roughly every 28 days.

SEX AND LOVE

The menopause means the end of the process of maturation of eggs. Ovulation stops. The eggs which are not utilized are reabsorbed into the body.

• • • • •

Puberty in boys is also triggered by the pituitary gland, which stimulates the testes to start releasing testosterone. Testosterone is the male sex hormone responsible for the changes in a boy's body. He begins the process of becoming a man.

Testosterone is made in the testes and controls sperm production. Unlike the eggs in women, which are there from birth, sperm are produced on an ongoing basis in the testes, right throughout a man's life, beginning at puberty. Because sperm can't form properly at body temperature, the testes are contained in the scrotum, a sort of bag of skin, which hangs outside the body. The sperm then go into a tube at the back of each testis called the epididymis to mature. The epididymis is a sort of coiled tube which would be about six metres long if it were unfurled.

During ejaculation, muscles contract to squeeze the sperm through the sperm duct, which runs from the testes into the penis, or more precisely into the urethra. The urethra is also the channel which carries urine from the bladder down the penis. Once the penis is erect, the mucles at the entrance of the bladder contract, preventing urine exiting, or semen entering, the bladder itself.

PHYSICAL CHANGES

En route from the testes to the penis, the sperm are joined by semen, which contains a sugar which both nourishes and helps the mobility of sperm. This semen is produced by structures called seminal vesicles, vesicle being another word for sac or cavity. Secretions from the prostate gland also help make up the semen which accompanies the sperm. At this stage they are now in the urethra and on their way down the penis. The penis itself is already erect. The erection happens when blood fills its spongy erectile tissue.

During intercourse the sperm are ejaculated into the vagina.

Sperm not ejaculated are reabsorbed into the man's body.

• • • • •

Hormones released at the onset of puberty also bring about physical changes in teenagers' bodies.

Girls develop breasts and the darker skin around the nipple, the areola, gets wider and somewhat darker. The external sexual organs develop too. The pad of fat on the pubic bone, the mons pubis, becomes fatter and more prominent, and pubic hair starts growing. So does hair under the armpits, and the hips and thighs become more rounded. Internal sexual organs develop too. And girls suddenly grow taller. Perspiration can become a problem and so can oily skin. And of course they get their periods.

Boys get underarm hair, some pubic hairs, may perspire more and get spots too. The penis, testes and scrotum enlarge and change colour somewhat, chest and shoulders broaden, hair on arms and legs thickens and starts to grow on their faces, voices get deeper because the larynx has enlarged and hair appears on their chests. And, of course, they too grow tall.

Teenagers need to know that these changes take place at a different rate, and to a different extent, in each and every child. This is decided largely by heredity. Whatever way they look, whatever speed they develop at, is normal. They should stop worrying and wait it out. Parents have to keep telling them that.

EPILOGUE

FINDING YOUR WAY

When I was working on Dr Brian McCaffrey's psychiatric team in the Eastern Health Board in Dublin during the 1970s, we slowly began to realize that individual or even group therapy was not enough. There were too few of us. Anyway, by the time people came for help there was already a lot of hurt and distress in their lives, psychological damage which might have been avoided.

We went out into the community, gave talks, seminars and courses to anyone who would listen, parent and teacher associations, schools, women's clubs, mother and toddler groups, teenage clubs, voluntary community workers, the unemployed. We went everywhere where people were gathered.

We called it 'imparting skills to the community'. We thought we were telling people how to do it, how to be good parents, responsible teenagers, empathetic partners, psychologically minded adults, upbeat members of the community. We weren't of course. We didn't tell people how to do anything. It's not possible.

My father was straight and plain-speaking, tough, fair and very critical. My mother was - and is - a born diplomat. Whenever any domestic negotiations were needed, she was inevitably the one who carried them out. It was my mother who always had to phone the plumber when he failed to turn up to finish a job, or the garage who had serviced the car but omitted to do all the repairs my father had requested, or the family member who had invited them to some get-together which they didn't wish to attend.

My father recognized my mother's diplomatic talents, but still wanted her to do it his way. He would tell her to really give out, to be firm and insist on an instant response, or to give some far-fetched excuse as to why they were not joining his brother for dinner. If it were serious enough, he'd scribble notes to her while she negotiated on the phone. Sensible woman, she invariably ignored him.

All couples row about such things. All couples have to learn the lesson. Individuals have their own style, their own way of doing things, they can't be told exactly what to say, must be trusted with the task.

No one can tell you how to talk to your children about sexual love. There really is no recipe book for sex education. You can be encouraged to overcome embarrassment, or rather to see it as decorum, a certain shyness being natural and proper to the subject matter of sex. It can help to understand the importance of privacy. You can be informed about biology, gain the facts about sexually transmitted diseases, be given some insight into the nature of children's sexual pleasure.

Only you can decide what to do, what to say and when to say it. Sex education cannot be separated from a moral code, the do's and don'ts about sexual behaviour which you believe in. Nor can it be divorced from the social conventions within which you live.

Take masturbation. All children masturbate. They do it first when they're quite small, around two years of age. At this stage, obviously, ejaculation or vaginal secretions play no role. Children do find it pleasurable. It's very important that they are not reprimanded sharply. Their behaviour is quite innocent, intellectually, emotionally and physically. But parents' views differ sharply about how tolerant they should be. Would you take your two-year-old daughter's doll away if you saw her in bed pleasurably rubbing herself against it? Or would you creep quietly away? And how would you react if she did it during the day while sitting on the sofa?

All I can say is treat her gently. Don't make her frightened or disgusted with herself. She's an innocent child, taking innocent pleasure. The extent to which you allow her to continue, however, will depend on circumstances, and your own personal preferences about what you believe to be right and wrong.

Heading into puberty, children masturbate again. Now there's clearly a moral issue involved, since this is adult sexual behaviour, a subject matter about which all churches, or religions, have their teachings. I can tell you all children do it, virtually all anyway, that boys have 'wet' dreams, ejaculate during sleep and girls have involuntary orgasms, which they find pleasurable. I can also tell you that, in the interest of psychological health and emotional well-being, teens should not be made feel guilty or ashamed.

It seems sensible to help them limit the extent of self-pleasuring, since masturbation is a lonely occupation. It can also be a form of retreat from social contact for teens too shy to mix properly, not just with the opposite sex, but with friends. It can signal social isolation. Old-fashioned solutions such as sport, physical activity generally, a range of interests and companionship with friends and family generally still make sense. Lonely boys and girls sometimes masturbate as consolation. That same loneliness may also drive them into serious sexual involvement too early. Excessive guilt, however, makes later sexual relationships difficult.

Beyond that, there's nothing I can say to you. Your moral values will largely dictate how you handle teenage masturbation, and all the other moral and social issues your teens face.

FINDING YOUR WAY

As a team of professionals in the 1970s, talking to those parents, teachers, teenagers, community workers and support groups, what we did was impart knowledge. We offered insights. We created the opportunity for people to see things differently. We helped people to feel differently. At best, all any professional can do is attempt to enlighten.

Family situations vary widely. Even the simple suggestion that you should answer children's questions when they ask is problematic. The question could come when younger big ears are around, ready to ridicule their seriously questioning older brother. Or older ears, ready to ridicule the younger ones. You may just have had an appalling row with their dad and be so full of sorrow that you cannot concentrate.

Parents have to struggle with their own limitations. In that split second between impulse and action, civilization is born. We stay our hand, or more importantly our tongue, and thus pave the way for our children to have a happier and more enlightened upbringing. When we question our instinctive, automatic responses, we ensure, in a very real sense, that the sins of the fathers are not visited on our sons. Brought up in brutality, we can manage to bring our children up in relative gentleness. Treated with carelessness, we manage to take great care of them. Over-indulged, we ensure we show proper firmness. We do all that by hesitating a moment before we act, or speak. But those battles with ourselves are, by definition, individual. Everything we do as parents is some kind of compromise between the ideal and what we actually manage as individuals.

We've moved away from emotional and physical brutality. We've said no to the old authoritarian model of state and family. Instead we're pulling ourselves up by our own bootstraps, trying to create a different and more enlightened world. Social historians tell me this has been happening steadily since the First World War. I believe them. But it happened for me somewhere in the late 50s with rock and roll. Then the 60s and the Beatles, the miniskirt and hippy flower power, all ushered in a new era.

Parents today have to continue on the path of gentle democracy, but they also have to balance the early excesses. We threw out the baby with the bathwater. A little anyway.

When we dismantled authoritarian church, school, state and family structures, we ditched authority too, threw our wisdom as adults out the window. Parents have to haul it back in, exercise good authority, be authoritative with a gentle mind and heart.

That's hard work. It's easy to reach back to dogma, or to dodge through *laissez-faire*. It's difficult to make good decisions. That's your task. No one can tell you how to do it.

Psychological studies suggest that it doesn't really matter whether parents are conservative or liberal in their beliefs and methods of upbringing. All that's required is that they are consistent. Children need to know where they stand. They need to know what to expect, or more precisely, what is expected of them. In that way they are not made neurotic. They are not constantly confronted with the unexpected. They also have something solid against which to measure their own opinions, something firm with which they can either agree or disagree.

That's true. But it's not just dithering parents who cause anxiety in their children, or encourage them to constantly test the boundaries, not believing you when you say no and asking again and again and again for something they want. It goes much deeper. Children need authenticity. Teenagers in particular need their parents to be emotionally honest. Changing your mind is not what matters most. On the contrary, the ability to change your mind is essential if you are to learn anything, especially if you are to learn from your children, which all of us need to do.

Parents must have the courage to steer clear of trendiness, to tell their children what they really think, even when that is not popular. We may also have to stop them doing certain things we don't approve of, depending on how old they are. We do this in matters of manners, in our attitudes to their study habits, or how they should treat, say, other children with a handicap. Why should it be any different when it comes to sexuality?

SEX AND LOVE

Young girls go to discos in tiny minis, with bordello-style bodices or tank tops which barely cover their bosoms. Some wear high boots too. They dress in clothes which seem sexually explicit. I know they don't intend to send out serious sexual signals. What they are saying is 'look at me' rather than 'approach me sexually'. It's true that innocence of intent protects them, up to a point. It's true that young boys probably understand the language of the current dress code, don't see it as at all provocative. And it's entirely possible that I'm old fashioned. But I don't believe it's a good idea for young teenage girls to go out dressed the way they do. That doesn't mean I would necessarily stop a young daughter, although I do think I would try to modify how she dressed. I would tell her what I thought and felt. And I would try to explain.

We began wearing minis in the 60s. But we still operated in a society which held a consensus about sin and sex. It was, of course, changing. We were ushering in the permissive society. There were, however, very strong taboos about early sex, definite ideas about good girls and naughty girls, and there was still that common language between boys and girls when it came to saying no. If you talked about sin, it was understood. There was also a great social price to pay, unwed pregnant girls were harshly treated. No girl wanted that. No boy did either.

The girl in the mini as short as today's was somewhat protected by the culture she lived in. The signal sent by the mini was toned down, counteracted to some extent by the cultural conviction that early sex was not a good idea.

Girls live in a very different culture today. The signals sent out by their disco-style clothes could be taken at face value. And I'm not convinced that individual girls are now so self-assertive that they can constantly say 'no' without strong social norms to back them up. I think our daughters are under a lot of pressure to say yes.

Teenagers need to hear an honest voice. That voice is yours. Many parents will not agree with what I've just said. That's why it is not possible to fulfil your very real need to hear how, exactly, sex education should be properly conducted, what, exactly, you should say. Only you know that. There is truly no recipe book.

A final story about my son Alex.

When he and his best friend were around 12, they went through that awful stage of telling very inappropriate jokes, the ones we call sick jokes. At the dinner table one evening they told me one, in giddy giggling unison, about a woman having a miscarriage.

I was deeply offended. I thought of all the women I knew who had had miscarriages, and of all the sadness involved. The joke wasn't funny, it was tasteless and ignorant and crude and vulgar, that joke. I'm sure I told the two boys that in no uncertain terms, I don't remember. But I do remember then telling them the true story of a woman who lived nearby, who had longed for years to have a baby. She finally became pregnant, waited for a while until she was absolutely sure, went out to celebrate with her delighted husband, and three days later found herself bleeding, was rushed into hospital, but miscarried. She was devastated, her husband perhaps even more so. And, for the moment at least, they felt there was no hope left.

The two boys sat opposite me, the unshed tears making their big eyes lustre. The joking was over, at least for the moment.

Children are ignorant. How can they be otherwise, until they learn? Those two boys had no idea of what it might be like to lose a baby. To them, miscarriages were a legitimate subject for jokes. But children have big hearts. They have so much to deal with themselves emotionally that they are acutely tuned in to peoples' feelings, deeply moved by any story they hear, only too willing to be sympathetic.

Children, including our difficult teens, are benign. They are not hostile, not the enemy, not monsters. They want to get it right, to be on our side. Parents don't have to break down barred doors to teach their children about sexual love. They do have to bridge the gap of embarrassment, but that's different. Sitting on the other side of that gap are young human beings, willing to empathize with us, dying to have us help them

FINDING YOUR WAY

facing the emotional turmoil that only sexual love can bring, and in dire need of our wisdom.

Talk to them. Tell them stories. Some of the stories may be factual. Others may merely be the way you see things, one person's perspective, offered to your teens as something they can take or leave as they see fit. Others will be parables with a powerful moral punch. Your teens will be willing listeners.

My thanks to Kate Cruise O'Brien, for her careful and sympathetic editing. And for her enthusiam and support.

Thanks also to Sally Pilkington, my diligent proof-reader.

And to my mother, who endlessly listened.